A Needle in a Haystack: Looking for Gaps in Treatment and Education in Emergency Medicine

Guest Editors
Klaudiusz Nadolny
Department of Emergency
Medical Service
Silesian Academy in
Katowice
Katowice
Poland

Filip Jaskiewicz
Department of Emergency
Medical Services
Medical University of Lodz
Lodz
Poland

Editorial Office
MDPI AG
Grosspeteranlage 5
4052 Basel, Switzerland

This is a reprint of the Special Issue, published open access by the journal *Healthcare* (ISSN 2227-9032), freely accessible at: https://www.mdpi.com/journal/healthcare/special_issues/96W0KXELGI.

For citation purposes, cite each article independently as indicated on the article page online and as indicated below:

Lastname, A.A.; Lastname, B.B. Article Title. *Journal Name* **Year**, *Volume Number*, Page Range.

ISBN 978-3-7258-5751-7 (Hbk)
ISBN 978-3-7258-5752-4 (PDF)
https://doi.org/10.3390/books978-3-7258-5752-4

A Needle in a Haystack: Looking for Gaps in Treatment and Education in Emergency Medicine

Guest Editors

Klaudiusz Nadolny
Filip Jaskiewicz

MDPI

Basel • Beijing • Wuhan • Barcelona • Belgrade • Novi Sad • Cluj • Manchester

Contents

About the Editors

Klaudiusz Nadolny

Klaudiusz Nadolny is a Professor of medical sciences and health sciences, Director of the Regional Ambulance Service in Sosnowiec, and Head of the Department of Emergency Medical Service at the Faculty of Medical Sciences, Academy of Silesia in Katowice. He completed his undergraduate studies in Emergency Medical Services and obtained a master's degree in management, followed by postgraduate programs in Health Care Law, Human Resources Management in Health Care, and an MBA. His research focuses on emergency medicine, prehospital care, and the organization and quality of medical emergency systems. He is the author of more than 220 scientific publications, a reviewer for several international journals, and co-creator of the prospective SIL-ROSC registry and one of the initiators of the national POL-OHCA cardiac arrest registry. Professor Nadolny is also Deputy Editor-in-Chief of the journal *Emergency Medical Service* and an active member of several expert groups of the Polish Ministry of Health and the Centre of Postgraduate Medical Education. He has been recognized with the Blessed Gerard Award and the Honorary Badge of Merit for Health Care by the Minister of Health, as well as the Prime Minister's Award for outstanding scientific achievements. In 2024, he received an honorary doctorate (Doctor Honoris Causa) from the National Medical University in Ivano-Frankivsk, Ukraine.

Filip Jaśkiewicz

Filip Jaśkiewicz is the Head of the Department of Emergency Medical Services at the Medical University of Lodz, Poland. He holds a Ph.D. in medical sciences and combines his experience as a paramedic, academic teacher, and researcher in the field of emergency medicine and medical education. His professional interests include prehospital care, first aid education, and innovation in life-saving equipment. He is the founder of the "ECO CPR – Ecological Manikin for Resuscitation Training," which received the Outstanding International Invention & Innovation Award at IPITEX 2023 in Bangkok, Thailand, and the inventor of the Active Compression Treatment (A.C.T.) Bandage. He has twice been recognized with the Best Teacher Award by the Medical University of Lodz for excellence in education and student engagement. He is the author and co-author of several peer-reviewed publications and serves on the editorial boards of international journals in the fields of emergency medicine and public health. His research promotes educational and technological innovation that bridges the gap between training and clinical practice.

Preface

The Reprint "A Needle in a Haystack: Looking for Gaps in Treatment and Education in Emergency Medicine" was conceived to highlight the unique and multifaceted character of emergency medicine as a discipline that connects science, logistics, and human resilience. Emergency medicine operates under extreme time constraints, dealing with patients of all ages and pathologies, and demands rapid, evidence-based decisions that can determine life or death.

This Reprint was designed to inspire researchers and practitioners to address the less visible yet crucial challenges in emergency care—those "needles in a haystack" that often remain hidden between guidelines and real-world practice. It gathers studies and reflections from diverse international contexts, showing how clinical innovation, educational reform, and equitable access to emergency services can together enhance patient outcomes and system preparedness.

The Editors hope that this collection will serve not only scientists and clinicians, but also educators, policymakers, and students who seek to understand and strengthen the chain of survival. By bridging gaps between research and practice, this Reprint invites continued collaboration across disciplines to make emergency medicine more effective, inclusive, and sustainable.

Klaudiusz Nadolny and Filip Jaskiewicz
Guest Editors

healthcare

MDPI

Editorial

A Needle in a Haystack: Looking for Gaps in Treatment and Education in Emergency Medicine—Editorial

Filip Jaskiewicz [1,*] and Klaudiusz Nadolny [2,3]

1 Department of Emergency Medical Services, Medical University of Lodz, 90-419 Lodz, Poland
2 Department of Emergency Medical Service, Faculty of Medicine, Silesian Academy in Katowice, 40-555 Katowice, Poland; prrm.knadolny@interia.pl
3 Collegium Medicum, WSB University, 41-300 Dabrowa Gornicza, Poland
* Correspondence: filip.jaskiewicz@umed.lodz.pl

1. Introduction

When this Special Issue, "A Needle in a Haystack: Looking for Gaps in Treatment and Education in Emergency Medicine," was first announced, its aim was to highlight the unique nature of emergency medicine as a discipline. Emergency medicine addresses life-threatening conditions across all age groups and aetiologies, often under severe time constraints and with limited resources [1]. It spans the entire continuum of care—from first aid provided by bystanders to advanced, multi-speciality interventions in emergency departments—requiring not only clinical excellence but also well-coordinated logistics, education, and system-level solutions to ensure optimal patient outcomes [2].

As noted in the original call for papers, conducting research in this field presents significant methodological and organisational challenges. Despite technological advances and growing scientific interest, many clinical recommendations still rely on weak evidence or expert consensus rather than robust data [3,4]. Moreover, the diversity and complexity of emergency medicine leave important questions underexplored, contributing to persistent gaps between guidelines and real-world practice [5].

Emergency medicine is also strongly shaped by global challenges such as ageing populations, climate-related disasters, armed conflicts, and pandemics, all of which increase demands on prehospital and hospital systems [6,7]. Addressing these issues requires high-quality, context-sensitive research that can be translated into practice.

The purpose of this Special Issue was to encourage researchers to think "outside the box," address knowledge gaps through innovative study designs and generate evidence with clear implications for patient care. Now, after ten articles have been published, this editorial summarises their key contributions, extracts cross-cutting insights, and outlines priorities for future research, education, and system development in emergency medicine [8].

2. Overview of Contributions

(1) ""Even Though the System Had Failed Him His Entire Life, We Were Failing Him Yet Again": How Clinical, Welfare, and Penal Medicine Interact to Drive Health Inequities and Medical Moral Injury."

A case study from Los Angeles examines how penal medicine, welfare systems, and clinical care intersect to perpetuate health inequities for justice-involved patients with injection-drug-use-related infective endocarditis. Physician narratives highlight moral injury when institutional constraints prevent equitable care. The authors call for restorative justice programmes, expanded harm-reduction services (including in carceral settings), and explicit institutional protocols for managing structurally vulnerable patients (Contribution 1).

(2) "Assessment of the Severity of COVID-19 Based on Examination and Laboratory Diagnostics in Relation to CT Imagery—Single-Centre Study."

This observational study links admission findings to subsequent CT-assessed lung involvement in COVID-19 patients. Significant associations were found between initial BNP, HCO_3^-, and base excess levels and severity of lung involvement, suggesting that simple laboratory and clinical markers can guide early risk stratification before imaging results are available (Contribution 2).

(3) "Successful Intraosseous Adenosine for Termination of SVT in a 3.5-Year-Old—Case Report and Literature Review."

A case report is presented of a 3.5-year-old child with supraventricular tachycardia (SVT) who was successfully treated using intraosseous (IO) adenosine after failed vagal manoeuvres. Sinus rhythm was restored after the second dose without recurrence. The case underscores IO administration as a viable alternative when intravenous access is difficult in paediatric emergencies (Contribution 3).

(4) "CALL TO ECLS—Acronym for Reporting ECPR Candidates from Prehospital Setting to Destination Centres."

The CALL TO ECLS acronym was validated as a prehospital communication tool for patients considered for extracorporeal CPR. Expert surveys showed high clarity, utility, and importance (I-CVI 0.87–0.97; S-CVI-AVE > 0.9), though the limited response rate was acknowledged as a study limitation. The revised version added explicit guidance on recognising "signs of life" (e.g., ROSC, motor response) during CPR to improve decisional clarity (Contribution 4).

(5) "What Mistakes Can Be Made When Performing Electrical Cardioversion?—Analysis of Emergency Medical Team Performance during Championships"

An analysis of competition scenarios (2015 and 2019) demonstrated high accuracy in initial qualification for electrical cardioversion in unstable tachycardia but declining adherence with successive shocks—especially for the re-activating synchronisation mode and selecting appropriate energies—while safety measures remained consistent. The findings highlight the need for refresher training and cognitive aids under time pressure (Contribution 5).

(6) "The Role of Paramedics in Diagnosing Sandifer's Syndrome—Case Report"

A 7-week-old with seizure-like episodes was ultimately diagnosed with Sandifer's syndrome, a rare manifestation of GERD often misdiagnosed as epilepsy. This case illustrates paramedics' role in early recognition through careful history-taking and assessment, preventing unnecessary anti-epileptic treatments (Contribution 6).

(7) "Uterotonic Drugs in Prevention and Management of Postpartum Haemorrhage in Prehospital Deliveries—Systematic Review."

A systematic review identified only four eligible studies on prehospital use of uterotonic agents, despite postpartum haemorrhage being a leading cause of maternal mortality. The evidence gap highlights the need for standardised EMS protocols and further research on uterotonic availability, dosing, and outcomes in prehospital settings (Contribution 7).

(8) "Adult Triage in the Emergency Department: Introducing a Multi-Layer Triage System."

Greek emergency departments implemented a multi-layer triage system integrating elements of established triage frameworks and early-warning scores (ESI, NEWS, HEART). This system aims to reduce under-triage, improve prioritisation, and offer flexibility while maintaining structured, reproducible decision-making (Contribution 8).

(9) "Medical Students' Knowledge and Adherence to Paediatric Choking Rescue Manoeuvre Guidelines—Multicentre Study."

A multicentre survey across 12 universities in Canada, Libya, and Poland (290 analysed responses) revealed substantial variability in knowledge retention regarding paediatric choking management, including body positioning, blind finger sweeps, and post-event follow-up. The findings argue for standardised, evidence-based curricula in paediatric first aid (Contribution 9).

(10) "Management of Polytraumatised Patients: Challenges and Insights into Air Transfer."

Analysis of 77 polytrauma patients transported by air in Romania (mean age 17.3 years; 74% road traffic accidents; 2:1 male predominance) calls for prevention strategies tailored to patient profiles and better risk analysis protocols to guide decisions on air versus ground transport efficiency (Contribution 10).

3. Cross-Cutting Themes

- Skills and systems integration: Technical proficiency (e.g., cardioversion, IO drug delivery) must be reinforced by reliable communication tools (e.g., CALL TO ECLS) and decision frameworks (e.g., multi-layer triage).
- Standardisation vs. local adaptation: Evidence gaps in uterotonic access and choking management contrast with validated tools like CALL TO ECLS, illustrating where global standards versus local tailoring are appropriate.
- Equity and moral injury: Justice-involved care and maternal health gaps reveal how emergency systems can perpetuate inequities unless welfare support, harm-reduction, and clear clinical protocols are integrated.
- Prehospital criticality: From air transfer to obstetric haemorrhage, early decisions in EMS repeatedly shape downstream outcomes, supporting targeted investment in prehospital education and infrastructure.

4. Future Priorities

1. Curriculum harmonisation for paediatric emergencies with longitudinal skill-retention studies.
2. Tool implementation research linking CALL TO ECLS use to ECMO activation times and survival.
3. High-reliability training for cardioversion, airway management, and CPR choreography.
4. Prehospital obstetric care trials testing uterotonic access, dosing, and outcomes.
5. Transport modality research comparing air vs. ground transfer outcomes using functional metrics.
6. Equity-focused interventions addressing harm reduction, re-entry support, and moral injury metrics.

5. Conclusions

This Special Issue collectively demonstrates that addressing gaps in emergency medicine requires a systems-oriented approach, bridging education, clinical practice, policy, and research. By integrating validated communication tools, harmonising training curricula, and prioritising equity-focused interventions, healthcare systems can become more resilient and responsive to emerging threats. Future efforts should foster international collaboration through multicentre trials, global clinical registries, and cross-border training initiatives to ensure that evidence-based practices reach diverse healthcare settings. Such coordinated actions can accelerate progress toward reducing preventable deaths, strengthening preparedness for mass-casualty events, and embedding continuous quality improvement across the entire chain of survival.

Author Contributions: Conceptualization, F.J.; writing—original draft preparation, F.J.; writing—review and editing, F.J. and K.N.; supervision, K.N. All authors have read and agreed to the published version of the manuscript.

Conflicts of Interest: The authors declare no conflicts of interest.

List of Contributions:

1. Ganesh, S.S.; Joyner, K.B.; Samra, S.; Bluthenthal, R.N.; Schneberk, T.W. "Even Though the System Had Failed Him His Entire Life, We Were Failing Him Yet Again": How Clinical, Welfare, and Penal Medicine Interact to Drive Health Inequities and Medical Moral Injury. *Healthcare* **2024**, *12*, 1354. https://doi.org/10.3390/healthcare12131354.
2. Ilczak, T.; Skoczynski, S.; Oclon, E.; Kucharski, M.; Strejczyk, T.; Jagosz, M.; Jedynak, A.; Wita, M.; Ćwiertnia, M.; Jędrzejek, M.; et al. Assessment of the Severity of COVID-19 Based on Examination and Laboratory Diagnostics in Relation to CT Imagery—Single-Centre Study. *Healthcare* **2024**, *12*, 1436. https://doi.org/10.3390/healthcare12141436.
3. Zachaj, J.; Kręglicki, Ł.; Sikora, T.; Moorthi, K.; Jaśkiewicz, F.; Nadolny, K.; Gałązkowski, R. Successful Intraosseous (IO) Adenosine Administration for the Termination of Supraventricular Tachycardia (SVT) in a 3.5-Year-Old Child—Case Report and Literature Review. *Healthcare* **2024**, *12*, 1509. https://doi.org/10.3390/healthcare12151509.
4. Sanak, T.; Putowski, M.; Dąbrowski, M.; Kwinta, A.; Zawisza, K.; Morajda, A.; Puślecki, M. CALL TO ECLS—Acronym for Reporting Patients for Extracorporeal Cardiopulmonary Resuscitation Procedure from Prehospital Setting to Destination Centers. *Healthcare* **2024**, *12*, 1613. https://doi.org/10.3390/healthcare12161613.
5. Ćwiertnia, M.; Dutka, M.; Białoń, P.; Szlagor, M.; Stasicki, A.; Mikulska, M.; Hajduga, M.B.; Bobiński, R.; Kawecki, M.; Ilczak, T. What Mistakes Can Be Made When Performing the Electrical Cardioversion Procedure?—Analysis of Emergency Medical Team Performance during the Championships in Emergency Medicine. *Healthcare* **2024**, *12*, 1724. https://doi.org/10.3390/healthcare12171724.
6. Wójcik, M.; Krysiak, D.; Babik, P.; Suchanek, Ł.; Ćwiertnia, M.; Trojak-Piętka, J.; Kawecki, M.; Pollok-Waksmańska, W.; Mikulska, M.; Ilczak, T. The Role of Paramedics in Diagnosing Sandifer's Syndrome. *Healthcare* **2025**, *13*, 883. https://doi.org/10.3390/healthcare13080883.
7. Wiciak, H.; Strózik, M.; Smereka, J. Uterotonic Drugs in Prevention and Management in Postpartum Haemorrhage in Prehospital Deliveries—A Systematic Review. *Healthcare* **2025**, *13*, 976. https://doi.org/10.3390/healthcare13090976.
8. Tsiftsis, D.; Tasioulis, A.; Bampalis, D. Adult Triage in the Emergency Department: Introducing a Multi-Layer Triage System. *Healthcare* **2025**, *13*, 1070. https://doi.org/10.3390/healthcare13091070.
9. Bieliński, J.R.; Huntley, R.; Timler, D.; Nadolny, K.; Jaśkiewicz, F. Medical Students' Knowledge and Adherence to Paediatric Choking Rescue Manoeuvre Guidelines: A Multicentre Study of Medical Education Curricula. *Healthcare* **2025**, *13*, 1441. https://doi.org/10.3390/healthcare13121441.
10. Anghele, M.; Moscu, C.-A.; Dragomir, L.; Lescai, A.-M.; Anghele, A.-D.; Baltă, A.A.Ș. Management of Polytraumatized Patients: Challenges and Insights into Air Transfer. *Healthcare* **2025**, *13*, 2181. https://doi.org/10.3390/healthcare13172181.

References

1. Chan, T.C. Specialty Grand Challenge: Emergency Health Services. *Front. Disaster Emerg. Med.* **2023**, *1*, 1310474. [CrossRef]
2. Beeson, M.S.; Bhat, R.; Broder, J.S.; Gaeta, T.J.; Janssen, A.; Karl, E.R.; Lo, B.M.; Moll, J.; Oh, L.; Patel, V.; et al. The 2022 Model of the Clinical Practice of Emergency Medicine. *J. Emerg. Med.* **2023**, *64*, 659–695. [CrossRef] [PubMed]
3. Kim, E.; Mahajan, P.; Barousse, C.; Kumar, V.A.; Chong, S.L.; Belle, A.; Roth, D. Global emergency medicine research priorities: A mapping review. *Eur. J. Emerg. Med.* **2025**, *32*, 12–21. [CrossRef] [PubMed]
4. Cimino, J.; Braun, C. Clinical Research in Prehospital Care: Current and Future Challenges. *Clin. Pract.* **2023**, *13*, 1266–1285. [CrossRef] [PubMed]
5. Martin-Gill, C.; Brown, K.M.; Cash, R.E.; Haupt, R.M.; Potts, B.T.; Richards, C.T.; Patterson, P.D.; Prehospital Guidelines Consortium. 2022 Systematic Review of Evidence-Based Guidelines for Prehospital Care. *Prehosp. Emerg. Care.* **2023**, *27*, 131–143. [CrossRef] [PubMed]

6. Werner, K.; Kak, M.; Herbst, C.H.; Lin, T.K. Emergency care in post-conflict settings: A systematic literature review. *BMC Emerg. Med.* **2023**, *23*, 37. [CrossRef] [PubMed]
7. Kolb, L.M.; Peters, G.A.; Cash, R.E.; Ordoobadi, A.J.; Castellanos, M.J.; Goldberg, S.A. Prehospital care for traumatic brain injuries: A review of U.S. state emergency medical services protocols. *Am. J. Emerg. Med.* **2024**, *84*, 158–161. [CrossRef] [PubMed]
8. Bai, E.; Zhang, Z.; Xu, Y.; Luo, X.; Adelgais, K. Enhancing prehospital decision-making: Exploring user needs and design considerations for clinical decision support systems. *BMC Med. Inform. Decis. Mak.* **2025**, *25*, 31. [CrossRef] [PubMed]

healthcare

MDPI

Article

Management of Polytraumatized Patients: Challenges and Insights into Air Transfer

Mihaela Anghele [1,2], Cosmina-Alina Moscu [1,2,*], Liliana Dragomir [1,2], Alina-Maria Lescai [1,2,*], Aurelian-Dumitrache Anghele [1] and Alexia Anastasia Ștefania Baltă [1,2]

1 Faculty of Medicine and Pharmacy, "Dunărea de Jos" University of Galați, 800008 Galați, Romania; anghele.mihaela@yahoo.com (M.A.); lilianadragomir2017@gmail.com (L.D.); anghele_aurelian@yahoo.com (A.-D.A.); alexiabalta@yahoo.ro (A.A.Ș.B.)

2 "St. Apostle Andrei" Clinical Emergency County Hospital, 800578 Galați, Romania

* Correspondence: cosmina_caluian@yahoo.com (C.-A.M.); alina.lescai@ugal.ro (A.-M.L.)

Abstract: Background and Objectives: Despite the potential benefits for the patient, aerospace interventions pose significant risks. Pre-hospital triage and patient transport are two essential elements for achieving an organized system of trauma. The advantages and disadvantages of using land transport from the scene of the accident to the trauma centers have been extensively studied, but there are gaps for air transport, and their exact level of efficiency is not known. Materials and Methods: The present study includes a total number of 77 patients, present at SMURD Galați air service for polytraumas caused by various mechanisms, with pluri-regional involvement. The identification of patients, as well as the selection of the most important anamnestic data, was performed after signing a confidentiality agreement; subsequently, all this information was introduced in centralized tables made in the statistical program IBM SPSS Statistics V24. Results: Out of the total of 77 polytraumatized patients who needed air transfer, an average age of 17.3 years will be noted, with a predominance of males in a 2:1 ratio. Most polytraumas are due to road accidents (74%) and patients with minimal tri-regional damage (51.4%). Conclusions: Taking into account the existing statistics in this research, it is important to implement prevention elements, designed based on the profile of the polytraumatized patient. Thus, accessing the most important characteristics of these patients can be an extremely important starting point in reducing the incidence of polytrauma or even patient deaths.

Keywords: polytrauma patient; car crash polytrauma; more than three regions affected by polytrauma

1. Introduction

Air ambulances are an integrated component of modern care for traumatic pathologies. They are able to transport patients to facilities with higher capacities, to extract injured patients from hostile terrain, and to transport them quickly to a trauma center [1].

Pre-hospital triage and patient transport are two essential elements for achieving an organized system of trauma. Current studies do not clearly define the benefits of helicopter transport over mortality in a prehospital trauma system with medical staff [2].

Recent research has provided evidence supporting broader assumptions about air transport efficiency. This demonstrates that air transport does not reduce the total time required to transport a patient, but reduces the time spent by the patient between medical units [1]. As a general conclusion, these studies demonstrated the importance of factors with the potential to influence patients' conditions. Key influencing factors include the availability of advanced interventions, qualified staff, prompt service, and access to specialized trauma centers [3].

While air medical transport offers notable clinical advantages, it is also associated with distinct operational risks. Adverse weather conditions, limited visibility, and night-time operations can compromise both safety and mission effectiveness. Consequently, the decision to deploy air ambulances must be guided by a balanced consideration of clinical urgency and operational safety constraints [4,5].

Although air transport may not significantly reduce the total transport time, it plays a crucial role in shortening the time required to access specialized trauma centers, especially during inter-facility transfers. Also, recent studies have shown that the presence of a doctor during helicopter transfer improves patient outcomes [5–7].

For this reason, although the air transport of patients has been widely available for several decades, it is still used with great caution (the benefits of this still require more extensive studies).

The benefits associated with air transport by helicopter are influenced by many variables specific to each mission and include the severity of injuries, their mechanism of production, the ability to transport patients from hard to reach or long distances, and specific transport algorithms [4]. While land transport has been widely studied, the efficiency of air transport in trauma cases remains uncertain and under-researched [6,8].

Since 1997, Mobile Emergency Service for Resuscitation and Extrication (S.M.U.R.D.), an institution that is intended to rescue critically ill patients, has been carrying out emergency aero-medical interventions and, in Romania, air rescue activity has been carried out by it since 2004 [9].

This service is a public one, regulated by the Government Emergency Ordinance no. 126/2003 on the operation, functioning, and financing of emergency assistance and was provided with helicopters purchased by the Ministry of Health and distributed to medical operators Fundeni Clinical Institute and Targu Mures County Emergency Clinical Hospital, by order of the Minister of Administration and Interior and the Minister of Health no. 277/777/2004 for the approval of the methodological norms for the application of GEO no. 126/2003 [9].

S.M.U.R.D. rescue missions are carried out with the light multifunctional Eurocopter EC 135 helicopter, equipped with the Special Aviation Unit of the Ministry of Internal Affairs and Administrative Reform. In the context of the Romanian S.M.U.R.D. aeromedical service, primary missions are direct interventions at the scene of an accident in order to stabilize and transport the patient to a medical center, while secondary missions involve the inter-clinical transfer of critical patients between health facilities in order to rapidly access specialized or higher level medical services [9].

Research on patient air transport has been limited to specific pathologies, so no general guideline has been developed to facilitate the choice of the most appropriate mode of transport, nor the definition of over-triage when the helicopter is used to perform those inter-clinical transfers [6,8].

Considering the local specificity and the available resources, the aim of this study is to characterize the clinical and demographic profile of polytraumatized patients transported by air by the S.M.U.R.D. Galați service, as well as to analyze the main interventions applied during the transfer. The study aims to provide descriptive data useful for improving the organization of aeromedical transport services, especially in regions with limited access to trauma centers.

Although a direct comparison with land transport cannot be made due to the lack of a control group, we hypothesize that air transfer provides operational and logistical benefits in accessing specialized care for polytrauma cases, particularly in geographically isolated areas. However, due to the lack of complete and standardized data on transport duration and clinical outcomes (e.g., survival and hospitalization length), our analysis is limited to clinical and operational aspects observed during the transfer.

2. Material and Methods

The present study includes a database consisting of a total of 77 patients (young adults and pediatric patients), known to have multiple injuries through various mechanisms of production that required transport by air ambulance. The study is retrospective, as the information about the subjects was collected over 5 years, between 2015 and 2019. During the analyzed period, the SMURD Galați air ambulance service conducted a total of 1534 missions, distributed annually in a relatively balanced manner, with a peak in 2018 and a slight decrease in 2019, as illustrated in Figure 1.

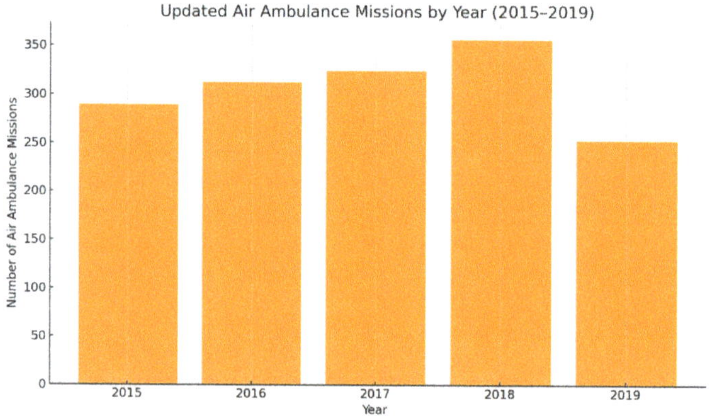

Figure 1. Update of air ambulance missions by year (2015–2019).

The inclusion criteria were patients with multiregional polytrauma, transported by the S.M.U.R.D. Galați air service between 2015 and 2019, and with complete medical data available. Exclusion criteria were as follows: patients with incomplete data, patients transported terrestrially, or cases with isolated trauma not requiring complex management. Parameters analyzed included demographics (age, sex), mechanism of trauma, Glasgow Coma Score (GCS), respiratory rate, ventricular rate, oxygen saturation (SpO_2, interventions applied (oxygen administration, artificial ventilation, intubation, RSI, cardiac massage), location of injuries, number of regions affected and type of mission (primary, secondary). Data were sorted and filtered according to clinically and statistically relevant criteria, but no information was collected on transport duration, survival, or length of hospitalization, which are proposed for future prospective research.

The data obtained from the research of the patient observation sheets were introduced in the statistical analysis program (IBM Statistics V. 24 *SPSS, Inc., Chicago, IL, USA) and Excel 2019, subsequently being filtered and sorted according to different criteria. Initially, the gross descriptive statistical parameters were calculated for all the variables for which this type of calculation approach was considered potentially useful. These include mean value, standard deviation (SD), minimum and maximum value for continuous numerical variables, frequency for categorical ones, median and mode value, and skewness and kurtosis indices. From a descriptive point of view, the corresponding diagrams were used for the graphical representations, using the software applications dedicated to the programs.

Categorical values were entered in the contingency tables and the non-parametric chi-square test (χ^2) was applied. For the calculation of the central trend and data dispersion, descriptive statistics were used, using the 95% confidence interval (confidence interval,

95%), the standard error of the mean, and the minimum and maximum value. For each of the existing statistical tests, a level of statistical significance for values of 0.05 was used, being calculated by the value of the *p*-index at two ends. Student's t-test was used to highlight the statistically significant differences between the groups or subgroups generated within the study group.

No information was collected on transport duration, time from incident to arrival of medical personnel, survival, or hospitalization length. These limitations are due to inconsistent or missing documentation in retrospective records and are acknowledged as critical aspects to be addressed in future research.

3. Results

The character of the missions of the SMURD crew is as follows: in a proportion of 59.7%, the mission has a primary character, followed by the missions with secondary character (29 patients, 37.7%). The smallest weights are represented in a proportion of 2.6% by special/rescue missions.

This section presents the findings of an analysis of 77 polytrauma patients transported by air ambulance. These findings are derived from a detailed examination of patient demographics, injury mechanisms, vital parameters, and statistical correlations, offering insights into the challenges and complexities of managing polytrauma cases.

3.1. Demographics and Injury Mechanisms

Out of the 77 patients, the majority were male (66.2%, $n = 51$), with a male-to-female ratio of 2:1. Figure 2 shows the distribution of patient ages. The average age was 17.3 years (±8.52), with notable peaks around 10 and 25 years. Most injuries (74%) were caused by road traffic accidents, encompassing drivers, passengers, and pedestrians. Additionally, 13% of injuries resulted from falls, while 11.7% were attributed to mechanisms such as crushing or physical aggression.

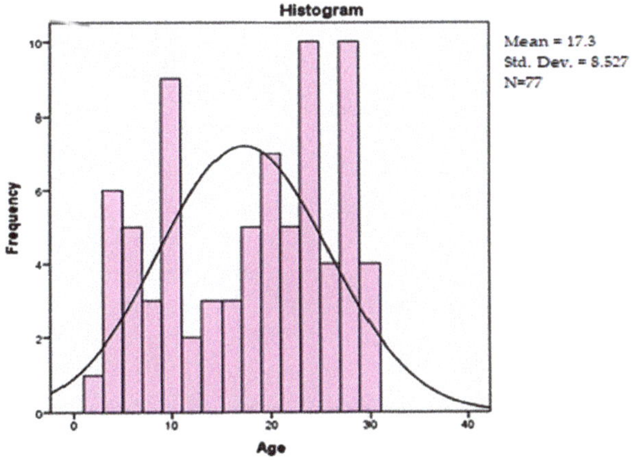

Figure 2. Age distribution of polytrauma patients transported by air ambulance (n = 77).

3.2. Patterns of Injury and Severity

Injury localization analysis showed that 51.9% of patients presented with tri-regional trauma, with a predominance of thoracic injuries (52%), followed by injuries to the limbs (45.5%) and spine (32.5%). Head injuries were reported in 19.5% of patients, abdominal injuries in 13%, and other injuries accounted for 6.5%. The percentage distribution of these categories is illustrated in Figure 3, where the vertical axis expresses the proportion (%) of the total 77 patients included in the study.

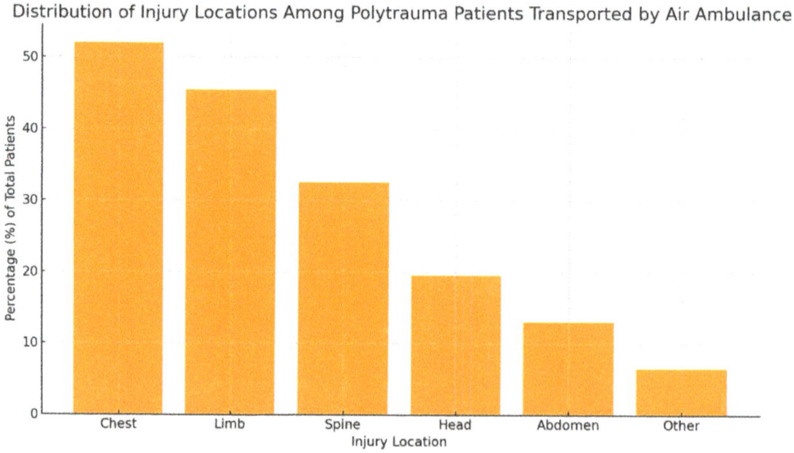

Figure 3. Distribution of injury locations among polytrauma patients transported by air ambulance.

3.3. Clinical Parameters and Interventions

The main clinical parameters are summarized in Table 1.

Table 1. Descriptive statistics of clinical parameters.

	N	Range	Minimum	Maximum	Mean	Std. Deviation	Skewness		Kurtosis	
							Statistic	Std. Error (Skew.)	Statistic	Std. Error (Kurt.)
GCS Scale	77	12	3	15	10.82	5.253	−0.631	0.274	−1.485	0.541
Respiratory Rate	77	20	0	20	9.91	7.499	−0.387	0.274	−1.498	0.541
Ventricular Rate	77	161	0	161	95.6	35.09	−0.961	0.274	1.666	0.541
SpO_2 (Oxygen Saturation)	77	100	0	100	90.95	24.479	−3.437	0.274	10.455	0.541
Systolic BP (mmHg)	77	120	70	120	108.7	22.6	−0.45	0.274	−0.28	0.541

The results of the Glasgow Coma Scale (GCS) scores ranged from 3 to 15, with an average value of 10.82 and a standard deviation of 5.25. The values of skewness and kurtosis indicate a homogeneous distribution. Respiratory rate analysis showed an average value of 9.91 breaths per minute, with a standard deviation of 7.499 breaths per minute. The ventricular rate exhibited a maximum value of 161 bpm, with an average of 95.60 bpm and a standard deviation of 35.09 bpm.

Oxygen saturation levels ranged widely, with a mean value of 90.95% and a maximum of 100%. The highest values were recorded after medical interventions during air transfer. Upon arrival at the scene or during initial evaluation, several patients presented with moderate to severe hypoxemia. Consequently, oxygen supplementation was required in 68.8% of cases, most frequently via simple mask or assisted ventilation, to stabilize respiratory function before or during transfer.

Among the 77 patients included in the study, 12 individuals (15.6%) were identified as hypotensive at the time of initial assessment, defined by a systolic blood pressure below 90 mmHg. All hypotensive patients required oxygen supplementation, while 75% ($n = 9$) underwent rapid sequence induction (RSI) for airway management. Endotracheal intubation was successfully performed in six of these cases. All hypotensive patients received intravenous crystalloid fluids, and vasopressor therapy was initiated in three cases to manage persistent hypotension. No patients received blood products, tranexamic acid (TXA), fibrinogen, or invasive monitoring, reflecting the logistical limitations and emergency protocols applicable during air transfer. Intravenous fluid resuscitation with crystalloids was administered in all 12 patients. Additionally, vasopressor therapy was initiated in three cases to manage persistent hypotension. This subgroup exhibited significantly lower Glasgow Coma Scale (GCS) scores, necessitating immediate stabilization measures during air transport.

Of the total group analyzed, only 3 subjects presented cardiac arrhythmias: 2 patients (2.6%) experienced tachycardia, while 1 patient (1.3%) experienced asystole. Additionally, one patient (1.3%) presented with severe mixed dyspnea.

Of the total patients analyzed, 68.8% required oxygen administration during air transfer, of which, 35.1% received oxygen by simple mask. A total of 19.5% required artificial ventilation, defined in this context as assisted ventilation by devices such as bag-valve-mask (BVM) in the absence of intubation. Orotracheal intubation was performed in 6.5% of patients, while the Rapid Sequence Intubation (RSI) protocol was initiated in 20.8% of patients. However, orotracheal intubation was completed in only 6.5% of cases due to various clinical reasons, including patient instability, spontaneous recovery of respiration, or constraints related to the limited duration of transfer. No supraglottic airway devices (such as laryngeal mask airways) were recorded in the documentation, which may reflect equipment availability or crew preference during the analyzed missions. It should be noted that RSI was applied as a preparatory measure for intubation by administering sedatives and muscle relaxants, but not all of these cases were completed with endotracheal intubation due to various clinical reasons (instability, spontaneous breathing recovery, or constraints related to the duration of transfer). Also, 2.6% of patients required external cardiac massage.

3.4. Statistical Correlations and Observations

Statistical analyses revealed significant relationships between two scalar variables: age (in years) and GCS scores. Figure 4 illustrates the graphical representation of the linear regression analysis between these variables, which provides the potential to make predictions. The regression equation indicates a weak positive correlation ($R^2 = 0.060$), meaning that only a small portion of GCS variation is explained by age. This suggests that only 6% of the variation in GCS scores can be attributed to age, highlighting a limited dependency. The scatter plot shows variability, particularly among younger patients with lower GCS scores, reflecting the severity of their neurological impairment.

In addition, Table 2 displays the results of a paired-samples t-test conducted to evaluate the differences between the two variables. The test revealed a statistically significant mean difference of 6.481 ($p < 0.001$) between age and GCS scores, with a 95% confidence interval ranging from 4.472 to 8.489. These findings emphasize the systematic disparity between the two variables, demonstrating that younger patients are more likely to have lower GCS scores, indicative of greater trauma severity.

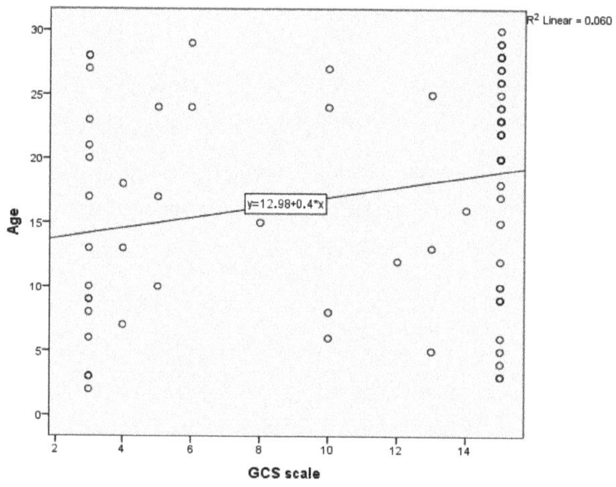

Figure 4. Correlation between Glasgow Coma Scale (GCS) and age.

Table 2. Paired *t*-test results comparing age and GCS.

	Mean	Std. Deviation	Std. Error Mean	95% Confidence Interval (Lower)	95% Confidence Interval (Upper)	T	Df	Sig. (2-Tailed)
Age–GCS Scale	6.481	8.848	1.008	4.472	8.489	6.427	76	0

In the following, we tried to find statistically significant correlations to highlight the relationships of dependence or even causality between individual variables. Thus, the first intention ANOVA testing was performed to quantify the degree of dependence of patients' age (as a scalar variable, dependent) in relation to the mechanisms of production or the number of affected regions. Thus, it was observed that between age and the mode of production of polytrauma there is no statistically significant correlation according to the ANOVA test (Levene = 0.410, ANOVA = 0.452). The same situation is encountered in the case of the interaction of this scalar variable in relation to the number of affected regions, no statistically significant correlation being demonstrated (Levene = 0.986, sig. ANOVA = 0.679).

Pearson index bivariate correlations were used for continuous variables. They did not detect any statistically significant correlations except for those between the mechanism of polytrauma production and the need for oro-tracheal intubation (sig = 0.038) as shown in Table 3.

Table 3. Pearson correlation between polytrauma variables and emergency response measures.

	Mechanism of the Polytrauma	Number of Regions Affected	Localization of the Polytrauma	Arrhythmias	Dyspnea	Oxygen	Intubation	External Cardiac Massage	Extrication	Restraint
Mechanism of the polytrauma	1	0.028	−0.127	0.216	−0.062	0.001	−0.237 *	−0.088	0.189	−0.207
Number of regions affected	0.028	1	0.552 **	0.093	0.152	0.12	0.131	0.11	−0.001	0.34
Localization of the polytrauma	−0.127	0.552 **	1	0.075	0.098	0.051	0.181	0.085	0.03	0.087

* Correlation is significant at the 0.05 level (2-tailed). ** Correlation is significant at the 0.01 level (2-tailed).

3.5. Comparative Outcomes by Injury Mechanism

The information presented above (Table 4) is analyzed below, by descriptive statistics, by performing independent t-tests. Thus, two groups of patients were created by reference to the mechanism of polytrauma production, as follows: those who were victims of road accidents (57 patients of sublot A), respectively, and polytraumas due to other causes (20 patients of sublot B). The t-test results revealed significant differences, particularly regarding intubation needs and average age between subgroups A and B.

Table 4. Independent samples test.

Variable	Levene's Test F	Sig.	T	Df	Sig. (2-Tailed)	Mean Difference	Std. Error Difference	95% CI Lower	95% CI Upper
GCS scale	0.543	0.464	−1.223	75	0.225	−1.664	1.361	−4.375	1.047
			−1.221	33.208	0.231	−1.664	1.363	−4.436	1.107
Oxygen	0.15	0.699	−0.213	75	0.832	−0.074	0.346	−1.736	1.588
			−0.211	32.661	0.834	−0.074	0.35	−0.786	0.638
Intubation	19.91	0	1.974	75	0.052	0.286	0.145	−0.003	0.575
			2.67	66.113	0.01	0.286	0.107	0.072	0.5
External cardiac massage	3.051	0.085	0.842	75	0.403	0.035	0.042	−0.048	0.118
			1.427	56	0.159	0.035	0.025	−0.014	0.084

The GCS score (average age for polytraumas due to road accidents was 10.39 points, respectively, 12.05 points for the other sublot). Although the significant value according to the t-test of the equivalence of the averages is 0.225, it can be concluded that at the level of the group there were lower GCS scores in the case of polytraumas from sublot A.

There was a lack of statistically significant differences between the two sublots, in relation to the need for oxygen (sig = 0.832) or performing cardiac massage to stabilize the patient during the transfer (sig = 0.403).

In the case of intubations performed during the transfer, the existence of significant differences between the two sublots can be observed (sig of the Levene test less than 0.01, respectively, sig of the t-test of the equivalence of the averages of 0.01). For this reason, we reject the null hypothesis and admit that, in the case of the group analyzed in the present research, there are differences between sublots A and B in terms of trachial intubation and average age.

In Table 5 is presented a descriptive statistic of the different variables analyzed in this research, depending on the mechanisms of polytome production, being associated with the significant values according to the Chi square tests. The only variables between which significant differences were defined (sig = 0.000) are represented by the production mechanisms and the location of the affectation. Thus, it is noted that, in road accidents, the association of regions is present, while in polytraumas by fall the cephalic extremity is predominantly affected, and in polytraumas by other mechanisms, thoracic injuries is predominant.

Table 5. Descriptive statistics and chi-square analysis of clinical variables by mechanism of polytrauma.

		Car Crash		Fall		Other Mechanism		Simulation Exercise		Chi Square Test Sig.
		Count	Column Valid *n*%	Count	Column Valid *n*%	Count	Column Valid *n*%	Count	Column Valid *n*%	
Localization of the trauma	Head trauma	0	0	1	10	0	0	0	0	0.00
	Chest trauma	2	3.6	0	0	2	22.2	0	0	
	Abdomen trauma	1	1.8	0	0	0	0	0	0	
	Pelvis trauma	1	1.8	0	0	0	0	0	0	
	Lim injury	7	12.5	0	0	2	22.2	0	0	
	Association of areas affected	45	80.4	9	90	5	55.6	0	0	
	Simulation exercise	0	0	0	0	0	0	1	100	
Number of region affected	1 region affected	6	10.5	0	0	3	33.3	0	100	0.00
	2 regions affected	12	21.1	4	40	1	11.1	0	0	
	3 region affected	8	14	1	10	1	11.1	0	0	
	>3 region affected	31	54.4	5	50	4	44.4	0	0	
	Simulation exercise	0	0	0	0	0	0	1	100	
Sex	M	36	63.2	8	80	6	66.7	1	0	0.66
	F	21	36.8	2	20	3	33.3	0	0	
Oxygen	Mask	20	35.1	4	40	3	33.3	0	0	0.277
	Ambu Bag	6	10.5	0	0	0	0	0	0	
	No	15	26.3	2	20	6	66.7	1	100	
	Ventilator	13	22.8	2	20	0	0	0	0	
	Taken into in-tub	3	5.3	2	20	0	0	0	0	
Intubation	No	39	68.4	8	80	9	100	1	100	0.534
	With induction	14	24.6	2	20	0	0	0	0	
	Without induction	4	7	0	0	0	0	0	0	
External cardiac massage	No	55	96.5	10	100	9	100	1	100	0.888
	Yes	2	3.5	0	0	0	0	0	0	
Defibrillation	No	57	100	10	100	9	100	1	100	0.352
	Yes	0	0	0	0	0	0	0	0	
Extrication	No	54	94.7	9	90	7	77.8	1	100	
	Yes	3	5.3	1	10	2	22.2	0	0	

4. Discussions

The results of this study provide detailed insights into the characteristics of polytrauma patients transported by air, as well as the interventions applied. When compared to the literature, the findings align with international observations, highlighting the challenges and benefits of this type of transport.

4.1. Demographic Profile and Trauma Mechanisms

Of the 77 patients analyzed, 66.2% were male, with a mean age of 17.3 years. This result is consistent with other studies that identify young males as the group at highest risk of severe polytrauma, especially due to their involvement in risky behaviors, such as aggressive driving or playing dangerous sports [10,11].

The distribution of trauma mechanisms shows that road traffic accidents were the main cause (74%), followed by falls (13%) and other mechanisms, such as physical assaults (11.7%).

These patterns align with established findings in the literature, indicating that high-energy trauma mechanisms, such as road traffic accidents, often result in injuries to the thoracic and extremity regions. Such injuries are frequently associated with significant morbidity and necessitate prompt and specialized medical intervention.

Although the database included both pediatric and adult patients, no statistical comparison was conducted between the two subgroups regarding injury mechanisms, injury types, or number of affected regions, due to the relatively small sample size and the skewed age distribution (mean age 17.3 years). This is acknowledged as a limitation.

These data are supported by Roshanaei et al. (2022), who identified road traffic accidents (39.6%) and falls (30.2%) as the predominant mechanisms of trauma among patients [12].

Similarly, Bradshaw et al. (2017) found that road traffic accidents and falls each accounted for 41% of pediatric trauma cases, highlighting variations between low- and high-income countries [13].

In contrast, in rural or mountainous areas, falls dominate as the main mechanism of injury, highlighting the importance of regional factors in determining trauma patterns [14].

Hulme (2015) supports this observation, noting that road traffic accidents and falls are the leading causes of death among children and adolescents in low- and middle-income countries [15].

These data also reflect the findings of Pascual-Marrero et al. (2018), who showed that road traffic accidents and falls are among the most common mechanisms of trauma, with a significant impact on morbidity and mortality in Puerto Rico [16].

In recent years, the effectiveness and outcomes of helicopter emergency medical services (HEMS) have been increasingly studied, particularly in trauma populations. For instance, Wejnarski et al. analyzed data from over 3000 patients with trauma or myocardial infarction transported by HEMS in Poland and reported significant differences in patient characteristics and types of missions compared to ground transport, underlining the strategic role of air transport in critical scenarios [17].

Similarly, Weinlich et al. evaluated over 1700 HEMS trauma cases in Germany and emphasized the added value of early intervention, advanced procedures, and shorter prehospital times, contributing to improved outcomes [18].

Our study shares similarities with these reports in terms of the predominance of trauma from road traffic accidents and the necessity for interventions such as oxygen administration and airway management. However, unlike these larger datasets, our cohort included a younger population (mean age 17.3 years), and procedures were adapted to the regional operational limitations and patient status during short transfers.

Moreover, Pham et al. found that faster on-scene times during HEMS missions were associated with reduced mortality in trauma patients, underscoring the critical importance of efficient scene management [19]. Although our study did not analyze scene times or patient outcomes, this highlights an important area for future prospective research.

Additionally, Lapidus et al. compared HEMS and road ambulance transports in Sweden and demonstrated superior survival rates in patients transported by helicopter, especially in rural or remote settings. These results suggest a potential benefit that may apply to systems like Romania's, particularly in regions with long distances to trauma centers [20].

Taken together, these studies support the growing consensus that HEMS offers a meaningful advantage in selected trauma cases. While our findings are primarily descriptive, they align with international trends and further emphasize the need to standardize data collection, incorporate outcome measures, and facilitate inter-center comparisons in future research.

4.2. Location and Severity of Injuries

The majority of patients in this study presented with tri-regional injuries (51.9%), with a predominance of thoracic, extremity, and spinal injuries. These findings align with studies by Chilvers et al. (2017), who demonstrated that high-energy trauma most frequently affects these regions, especially in road traffic accidents [21].

Multiple injuries carry a significant risk of complications, including multiple organ failure. Studies by Biewener et al. (2004) confirm that combined chest and extremity injuries are associated with higher rates of intraoperative and postoperative complications [5]. The findings of this study further support the need for rigorous protocols for the rapid assessment and intervention of patients with severe polytrauma.

4.3. Clinical Parameters and Emergency Interventions

Clinical parameters indicate moderate severity of trauma, with a mean Glasgow Coma Scale (GCS) score of 10.82. In the literature, patients with GCS scores below 10 are considered to be at high risk of mortality, underscoring the urgency of rapid interventions for these cases [22]. Studies suggest that lower GCS scores are associated with an increased likelihood of intubation and poorer outcomes, especially in patients with severe trauma [23]. Emergency interventions included oxygen administration (68.8%) and orotracheal intubation (20.8%). It should be emphasized that the reported 100% SpO_2 values reflect post-intervention measurements, not baseline saturation upon team arrival, thus supporting the necessity for oxygen therapy in a significant proportion of patients. Furthermore, the presence of hypotension in 15.6% of cases highlights the hemodynamic instability frequently encountered in polytrauma patients and reinforces the necessity for prompt and aggressive prehospital resuscitation strategies. These include early intravenous fluid administration, implementation of rapid sequence induction protocols, and definitive airway management to prevent further clinical deterioration during transfer. These data are comparable to those reported by Hoffmann et al. (2017), who highlighted that prehospital intubation was performed predominantly in patients with GCS ≤ 8, improving outcomes when combined with sedation [22]. Furthermore, McMullan et al. (2013) discussed the prevalence of prehospital oxygen use in trauma care, noting its critical role in cases of hypoxemia and hemorrhagic shock [24].

Patients with trauma also face a substantially elevated risk of venous thromboembolism, primarily due to prolonged immobilization and the physiological changes associated with severe injuries, as highlighted by Anghele et al. (2024) [25,26]. This underscores the need for vigilant monitoring and preventive strategies during both transport and hospitalization [25]. Additionally, the first 60 min post-trauma, often referred to as the "golden hour," are crucial for determining patient survival and long-term outcomes [26].

Significant psychological challenges, such as intrusive thoughts and stress, are also common in polytrauma patients, which can delay recovery even in cases of successful medical interventions [27]. These findings emphasize the need for an integrated approach that addresses both physical and psychological factors in trauma care [28]. Furthermore, significant differences between patients involved in motor vehicle crashes and those with injuries from other mechanisms highlight the importance of personalizing intervention protocols, given the variable severity of injuries [29].

4.4. Impact of the Medical Team on Prognosis

Our study highlights the constant presence of a doctor and a nurse in all air transfers, in contrast to other research. Dewhurst et al. (2001) demonstrated that the presence of qualified medical personnel, such as anesthesiologists, is essential for the management of high-risk patients, reducing the incidence of adverse events, which were reported in 12% of cases [30].

Recent studies highlight the essential role of air transportation in emergency medicine, emphasizing its potential to reduce time to specialized care and improve patient outcomes. However, our study did not evaluate transfer times, and these references are cited here only to provide context. The presence of specialized medical personnel on board, particularly in severe cases, further contributes to the optimization of clinical management, leading to a reduced risk of complications and short-term mortality [31,32].

However, the prolonged exposure of healthcare professionals, particularly those in emergency departments, to high-stress environments significantly impacts their mental health and performance, as noted by Moscu et al. (2023), emphasizing the need for targeted support systems to mitigate these effect [33]. Mulrooney (1991) further highlighted the importance of physicians adapting to the unique conditions of the air environment to maintain or improve the condition of patients during transfers [34]. Moreover, the concept of the mobile intensive care unit (MOBI), introduced by Icenogle et al. (1988), demonstrated that the transport of critically ill patients with comprehensive medical care could lead to positive outcomes without complications during long-distance transfers, underscoring the crucial role of a well-equipped and adequately staffed medical team [35].

4.5. Implications for National Trauma Treatment Policy

The findings of this study can significantly support the development of clearer national policies for managing polytrauma in Romania. By outlining a detailed demographic and clinical profile of patients transported by air, the research provides a valuable framework for public health authorities and emergency response policymakers.

In particular, identifying the predominance of road traffic accidents and multiregional injuries justifies the need to revise prehospital triage criteria for air transport, ensuring that helicopter use is based on clearly defined clinical indications and resource efficiency. This may help reduce unnecessary over-triage and better allocate costly aeromedical resources.

Furthermore, correlations between GCS scores and patient age could inform updates to intervention algorithms, particularly for pediatric trauma cases. The study also underlines the need to establish a national trauma registry, incorporating structured aeromedical data to enable real-time protocol monitoring and optimization.

These conclusions may guide the strategic development of standardized national protocols for air transfer, improved training programs for aeromedical teams, and targeted investments in regional heliport infrastructure to enhance trauma system responsiveness. International studies also support this need; Tsuchiya et al. (2016) showed improved survival in trauma patients transported by helicopter, reinforcing the urgency of developing structured criteria for air transport use [36].

4.6. Comparison with Other Air Transport Systems

Compared to international systems, such as the United Kingdom, which reported over 221,000 emergency air missions between 1987 and 2009 [1], the Romanian system has limited resources. However, recent initiatives, such as the heliport at the Bucharest University Emergency Hospital, have demonstrated increased efficiency, with over 550 lives saved in five years [37]. These examples highlight the importance of investing in infrastructure and expanding capacity to meet international standards.

4.7. Limitations and Future Prospects

This study has several significant limitations that should be considered when interpreting the results.

The relatively small sample size of 77 patients limits the robustness of the conclusions and their applicability to national or international settings. In addition, the collection of data from a single geographic region and the retrospective study design may introduce biases, such as reliance on accurate medical documentation and selection of patients for air transfer, which could overestimate the benefits or challenges of this type of transport.

A key limitation is the absence of a control group consisting of polytrauma patients transported by land. Although this restricts the ability to draw direct comparative conclusions, our hypothesis remains that air transfer provides significant clinical and operational benefits in managing complex trauma cases, especially in situations where land access is limited or delayed. In such contexts, air transport ensures faster access to specialized trauma care, potentially improving patient outcomes despite the inherent risks and logistical challenges.

Additionally, the study population consisted predominantly of young patients, which reflects the real-world demographic profile of air-transferred trauma cases in the analyzed region but limits the generalizability of findings to other age groups.

A major limitation of this study is the absence of data on time-sensitive variables such as duration of transport and time from accident to initial medical contact, as well as outcome measures such as survival and length of hospitalization. These factors are essential for assessing the true impact of air medical transport and should be included in prospective, multicentric studies.

Furthermore, important variables such as long-term outcomes, operational conditions, or quality of life parameters were not included in the analysis. Future research should adopt a prospective design, include larger samples from multiple regions, and integrate control groups for a detailed comparison between air and ground transfers, with the aim of developing standardized national guidelines and assessing the impact on clinical outcomes and patient quality of life.

5. Conclusions

The study confirms the complexity of air-transferred polytrauma cases and describes the demographic and clinical profile of patients transported by helicopter in a regional Romanian context. The predominance of male patients and mechanisms such as road traffic accidents highlight the vulnerability of younger populations involved in high-risk activities. Tri-regional injuries and moderate severity of trauma reflect the need for coordinated prehospital care. Interventions such as oxygen administration, assisted ventilation, and intubation in selected cases illustrate the critical role of appropriately trained medical teams in the air transfer setting. Although the study did not evaluate outcomes or transfer duration, these descriptive findings can contribute to future discussions on optimizing aeromedical response protocols for trauma patients.

Author Contributions: Methodology, M.A.; Software, C.-A.M.; Validation, L.D.; Data curation, A.A.Ș.B.; Writing—original draft, A.-M.L.; Project administration, A.-D.A. All authors have read and agreed to the published version of the manuscript.

Funding: This research received no external funding.

Institutional Review Board Statement: The study was conducted in accordance with the Declaration of Helsinki, and the protocol was approved by the Ethics Committee of the Clinical Emergency Hospital, Galati, Romania (project identification code: 7580/14.04.2021, approval date 5 March 2025).

Informed Consent Statement: All subjects provided informed consent for inclusion before they participated in the study.

Data Availability Statement: Data is contained within the article. Data is unavailable due to privacy or ethical restrictions, a statement is still required.

Conflicts of Interest: The authors declare no conflict of interest.

References

1. Ruskin, K.J. Helicopter air ambulance services. *Curr. Opin. Anaesthesiol.* **2019**, *32*, 252–256. [CrossRef]
2. Ageron, F.X.; Debaty, G.; Savary, D.; Champly, F.; Albasini, F.; Usseglio, P.; Vallot, C.; Galvagno, S.; Bouzat, P.; TRENAU Group. Association of helicopter transportation and improved mortality for patients with major trauma in the northern French Alps trauma system: An observational study based on the TRENAU registry. *Scand. J. Trauma Resusc. Emerg. Med.* **2020**, *28*, 35. [CrossRef]
3. Huo, Y.; Couzner, L.; Windsor, T.; Laver, K.; Dissanayaka, N.N.; Cations, M. Barriers and enablers for the implementation of trauma-informed care in healthcare settings: A systematic review. *Implement. Sci. Commun.* **2023**, *4*, 49. [CrossRef] [PubMed]
4. Hamman, B.L.; Cué, J.I.; Miller, F.B.; O'Brien, D.A.; House, T.; Polk, H.C., Jr.; Richardson, J.D. Helicopter transport of trauma victims: Does a physician make a difference? *J. Trauma* **1991**, *31*, 490–494. [CrossRef]
5. Biewener, A.; Aschenbrenner, U.; Rammelt, S.; Grass, R.; Zwipp, H. Impact of helicopter transport and hospital level on mortality of polytrauma patients. *J. Trauma* **2004**, *56*, 94–98. [CrossRef] [PubMed]
6. Di Rocco, D.; Pasquier, M.; Albrecht, E.; Carron, P.N.; Dami, F. HEMS inter-facility transfer: A case-mix analysis. *BMC Emerg. Med.* **2018**, *18*, 13. [CrossRef]
7. Karanicolas, P.J.; Bhatia, P.; Williamson, J.; Malthaner, R.A.; Parry, N.G.; Girotti, M.J.; Gray, D.K. The fastest route between two points is not always a straight line: An analysis of air and land transfer of nonpenetrating trauma patients. *J. Trauma* **2006**, *61*, 396–403. [CrossRef]
8. Galvagno, S.M., Jr.; Sikorski, R.; Hirshon, J.M.; Floccare, D.; Stephens, C.; Beecher, D.; Thomas, S. Helicopter emergency medical services for adults with major trauma. *Cochrane Database Syst. Rev.* **2015**, *2015*, CD009228. [CrossRef]
9. SMURD. Intervenții Aeromedicale-SMURD. Available online: http://smurd.ro/unitati/interventii-aeromedicale/ (accessed on 14 February 2021).
10. Tabatabaei, M.S.H.Z.; Baigi, V.; Zafarghandi, M.; Rahimi-Movaghar, V.; Valizade Hasanloei, M.A.; Piri, S.; Khavandegar, A.; Naghdi, K.; Salamati, P. Epidemiology of injuries among patients admitted to Imam Khomeini Hospital, Urmia, affiliated with the national trauma registry of Iran. *Front. Emerg. Med.* **2024**, 8. [CrossRef]
11. De Araújo Júnior, F.A.; Matsubara, A.; Pereira, L.; Schmidt, E.H.B.; Kondlatsch, G.L.S. Epidemiology of spinal cord injury in a reference trauma center in Curitiba (Paraná, Brazil). *Coluna/Columna* **2021**, *20*, 137–143. [CrossRef]
12. Roshanaei, G.; Khoshravesh, S.; Abdolmaleki, S.; Bathaei, T.; Farzian, M.; Saatian, M. Epidemiological pattern of trauma patients based on the mechanisms of trauma: Trends of a regional trauma center in Midwest of Iran. *BMC Emerg. Med.* **2022**, *22*, 210. [CrossRef]
13. Bradshaw, C.J.; Bandi, A.; Muktar, Z.; Hasan, M.A.; Chowdhury, T.; Banu, T.; Lakhoo, K.; Hailemariam, M.; Ngu, F.; Croaker, D.; et al. International study of the epidemiology of paediatric trauma: PAPSA research study. *World J. Surg.* **2017**, *41*, 3005–3014. [CrossRef] [PubMed]
14. Martínez Casas, I.; Amador Marchante, M.A.; Păduraru, M.; Fábregues Olea, A.; Nolasco, A.; Medina, J.C. Thorax trauma severity score: Is it reliable for patient's evaluation in a secondary level hospital? *Rev. Esp. Cir. Ortop. Traumatol.* **2016**, *60*, 119–126.
15. Hulme, P. Mechanisms of paediatric trauma at a rural hospital in Uganda. *Rural. Remote Health* **2015**, *10*, 1376. [CrossRef]
16. Pascual-Marrero, A.; Ramos-Meléndez, E.O.; García-Rodríguez, O.; Morales-Quiñones, J.E.; Rodríguez-Ortiz, P.G. Trauma epidemiology in Puerto Rico: In-hospital morbidity and mortality from 2002 to 2011. *Trauma* **2018**, *20*, 15–25. [CrossRef]
17. Wejnarski, A.; Leszczyński, P.; Świeżewski, S.; Podgórski, M.; Farkowski, M.M.; Sterliński, M.; Panczyk, M.; Gotlib, J.; Rabczenko, D.; Gałązkowski, R. Characteristics of aeromedical transport, both interhospital and directly from the scene of the incident, in patients with acute myocardial infarction or acute trauma between 2011–2016 in Poland: A case-control study. *Adv. Clin. Exp. Med. Off. Organ Wroc. Med. Univ.* **2019**, *28*, 1495–1505. [CrossRef] [PubMed]
18. Weinlich, M.; Martus, P.; Blau, M.B.; Wyen, H.; Walcher, F.; Piatek, S.; Schüttrumpf, J.P. Competitive advantage gained from the use of helicopter emergency medical services (HEMS) for trauma patients: Evaluation of 1724 patients. *Injury* **2019**, *50*, 1028–1035. [CrossRef] [PubMed]
19. Pham, H.; Puckett, Y.; Dissanaike, S. Faster on-scene times associated with decreased mortality in Helicopter Emergency Medical Services (HEMS) transported trauma patients. *Trauma Surg. Acute Care Open* **2017**, *2*, e000122. [CrossRef]
20. Lapidus, O.; Rubenson Wahlin, R.; Bäckström, D. Trauma patient transport to hospital using helicopter emergency medical services or road ambulance in Sweden: A comparison of survival and prehospital time intervals. *Scand. J. Trauma Resusc. Emerg. Med.* **2023**, *31*, 101. [CrossRef]

21. Chilvers, G.; Janjua, U.; Choudhary, S. Blunt cervical spine injury in adult polytrauma: Incidence, injury patterns and predictors of significant ligament injury on CT. *Clin. Radiol.* **2017**, *72*, 907–914. [CrossRef]
22. Hoffmann, M.; Czorlich, P.; Lehmann, W.; Spiro, A.S.; Rueger, J.M.; Lefering, R.; Trauma Register DGU of the German Trauma Society (DGU). The Impact of Prehospital Intubation with and Without Sedation on Outcome in Trauma Patients with a GCS of 8 or Less. *J. Neurosurg. Anesthesiol.* **2017**, *29*, 161–167. [CrossRef]
23. Al-Thani, H.; El-Menyar, A.; Latifi, R. Prehospital versus Emergency Room Intubation of Trauma Patients in Qatar: A-2-year Observational Study. *N. Am. J. Med. Sci.* **2014**, *6*, 12–18. [CrossRef]
24. McMullan, J.; Rodriquez, D.; Hart, K.W.; Lindsell, C.J.; Vonderschmidt, K.; Wayne, B.; Branson, R. Prevalence of prehospital hypoxemia and oxygen use in trauma patients. *Mil. Med.* **2013**, *178*, 1121–1125. [CrossRef]
25. Anghele, A.D.; Marina, V.; Dragomir, L.; Moscu, C.A.; Fulga, I.; Anghele, M.; Popescu, C.M. Artificial Intelligence Applied in Early Prediction of Lower Limb Fracture Complications. *Clin. Pract.* **2024**, *14*, 2507–2521. [CrossRef]
26. Anghele, M.; Marina, V.; Anghele, A.-D.; Moscu, C.-A.; Dragomir, L. Negative Factors Influencing Multiple-Trauma Patients. *Clin. Pract.* **2024**, *14*, 1562–1570. [CrossRef] [PubMed]
27. Anghele, M.; Marina, V.; Moscu, C.A.; Romila, A.; Dragomir, L.; Anghele, A.-D.; Lescai, A.-M. Use of the WBSI questionnaire in a study group of patients with polytrauma during the period 2015-2021. BRAIN. *Broad Res. Artif. Intell. Neurosci.* **2023**, *14*, 36–50. [CrossRef]
28. Anghele, M.; Marina, V.; Moscu, C.A.; Dragomir, L.; Anghele, A.D.; Lescai, A.M. Emotional Distress in a Patients Following Polytrauma. *J. Multidiscip. Healthc.* **2023**, *16*, 1161–1170. [CrossRef]
29. Choffat, C.; Delhumeau, C.; Fournier, N.; Schoettker, P. Effect of Pre-Hospital Intubation in Patients with Severe Traumatic Brain Injury on Outcome: A Prospective Cohort Study. *J. Clin. Med.* **2019**, *8*, 470. [CrossRef] [PubMed]
30. Dewhurst, A.; Farrar, D.; Walker, C.; Mason, P.; Beven, P.; Goldstone, J. Medical repatriation via fixed-wing air ambulance: A review of patient characteristics and adverse events. *Anaesthesia* **2001**, *56*, 882–887. [CrossRef]
31. Fromm, R.; Varon, J. Air medical transport. *Chest* **1993**, *104*, 989–993.
32. Trifan, A.L.; Dragomir, L.; Anghele, M.; Elkan, E.M.; Munteanu, S.; Moscu, C.; Stoian, V.I.; Telehuz, A.; Zlati, M.L.; Lungu, M.; et al. Assessment of Transportation by Air for Patients with Acute ST-Elevation Myocardial Infarction from Non-PCI Centers. *Healthcare* **2021**, *9*, 299. [CrossRef]
33. Moscu, C.A.; Marina, V.; Anghele, A.D.; Anghele, M.; Dragomir, L.; Ciubară, A. The Impact of Work-Related Problems on Burnout Syndrome and Job Satisfaction Levels among Emergency Department Staff. *Behav. Sci.* **2023**, *13*, 575. [CrossRef]
34. Mulrooney, P. Aeromedical patient transfer. *Aust. Fam. Physician* **1991**, *20*, 509–513.
35. Icenogle, T.; Smith, R.; Nelson, R.; Machamer, W.; Davis, B. Long-distance transport of cardiac patients in extremis: The mobile intensive care (MOBI) concept. *Am. J. Emerg. Med.* **1988**, *6*, 326–331.
36. Tsuchiya, A.; Tsutsumi, Y.; Yasunaga, H. Outcomes after helicopter versus ground emergency medical services for major trauma—Propensity score and instrumental variable analyses: A retrospective nationwide cohort study. *Scand. J. Trauma Resusc. Emerg. Med.* **2016**, *24*, 140. [CrossRef] [PubMed]
37. Capital. Responsibility Saves Lives: Five Years Since the Inauguration of the Heliport Funded by Maxbet at the Bucharest University Emergency Hospital. 2024. Available online: https://www.capital.ro/responsabilitatea-sociala-salveaza-vieti-cinci-ani-de-la-inaugurarea-heliportului-finantat-de-maxbet-la-spitalul-universitar-de-urgenta-bucuresti.html (accessed on 2 May 2025).

healthcare

MDPI

Article

Medical Students' Knowledge and Adherence to Paediatric Choking Rescue Manoeuvre Guidelines: A Multicentre Study of Medical Education Curricula

Jakub R. Bieliński [1], Riley Huntley [2], Dariusz Timler [1], Klaudiusz Nadolny [3,4] and Filip Jaskiewicz [1,*]

1 Emergency Medicine and Disaster Medicine Department, Medical University of Lodz, 90-419 Lodz, Poland; jakub.bielinski@umed.lodz.pl (J.R.B.); dariusz.timler@umed.lodz.pl (D.T.)
2 Faculty of Applied Science, School of Nursing, University of British Columbia, Vancouver, BC V6T 2B5, Canada; rileydj@student.ubc.ca
3 Department of Emergency Medical Service, Faculty of Medicine, Silesian Academy in Katowice, 40-555 Katowice, Poland; prrm.knadolny@interia.pl
4 Collegium Medicum, WSB University, 41-300 Dabrowa Gornicza, Poland
* Correspondence: filip.jaskiewicz@umed.lodz.pl

Abstract: Background/Objectives: Bystander first aid in paediatric choking is crucial. It ought to be universally comprehensible and backed up by evidence-based guidelines. However, there still are inconsistencies in guidelines worldwide. The objective of this research was to assess the knowledge of medical students on paediatric choking rescue manoeuvres and their educational backgrounds in order to evaluate the impact of differences in educational curricula. **Methods:** Medical students from a total of 12 universities across Canada, Libya, and Poland were surveyed online. The questionnaire assessed the respondents' experience, training, and knowledge in first aid regarding foreign body airway obstruction in infants and children. **Results:** Out of 324 responses, 290 were evaluated. Although the students studied in only 3 countries, they represented 37 countries of origin. A total of 7 new reference groups were created based on guideline identification. A comparison of 4 clinical scenario questions revealed that certain training providers communicate recommendations more effectively to medical students, as their guidelines seem to have better knowledge retention. **Conclusions:** There are important differences in medical student knowledge, possibly due to discrepancies in training programs and guidelines. Variability was found in body position, anti-choking suction devices, blind finger sweeps, and medical follow-ups. More research is needed to standardize training and improve worldwide choking management outcomes.

Keywords: first aid; paediatric; children; foreign body airway obstruction; choking; airway; back blows; chest thrusts; abdominal thrusts; Heimlich manoeuvre

1. Introduction

Foreign body airway obstruction (FBAO), commonly known as choking, is one of the leading causes of accidental paediatric death worldwide, with 75% of all FBAO cases occurring in children younger than 3 years old [1,2]. In developed countries, around 300 to 600 fatal accidents occur annually, but the situation is significantly more dire in underdeveloped countries, where fatalities occur at twice the rate [3–5]. Despite increasing recognition, there has been a steady rise in the frequency of paediatric FBAO over an extended period [5]. Additionally, recent research indicates that almost half of fatalities happen before the administration of any rescue interventions, indicating disregard in first aid recognition and management of choking or considerable delays in providing appropriate rescue manoeuvres [6,7].

Severe airway blockage may result in respiratory failure and cardiac arrest [8]. However, even in cases of partial blockage, life-threatening complications, such as airway swelling and inflammation, can arise from the delayed extraction of foreign objects [9]. Evidence suggests the high importance of early bystander intervention in reducing potential risks and averting fatal outcomes for paediatric FBAO incidents. Prompt, effective action by bystanders and medical personnel is critical in choking emergencies, with the potential to prevent deterioration and improve survival.

A key determinant in successfully assisting a choking child is the rescuer's level of first aid knowledge and skills [10,11]. Providers need a clear understanding of guidelines to deliver effective care. Disturbingly, evidence indicates a lack of widespread competence among the general population in dealing with paediatric FBAO [12,13]. Even among caregivers of children, there is a notable lack of knowledge, with some studies suggesting that only 5% to 30% of parents and teachers demonstrate adequate awareness of the problem [14–16].

Individuals who received first aid training show significantly greater knowledge than those without, with evidence suggesting that around half of those trained have knowledge and comprehension levels above the minimal level [13]. These findings suggest that healthcare professionals with comprehensive first aid training should possess the best understanding of critical lifesaving techniques, such as airway management, during choking incidents.

However, there is insufficient high-quality evidence to conclusively determine the level of knowledge and skills among healthcare providers who may provide care to children. According to current evidence, self-evaluations of paediatric residents in foreign body removal show a low level of competency, and this does not appear to improve over time with increasing work experience [17]. Prehospital emergency medical care personnel trained in basic life support, who are often called to paediatric emergencies, also demonstrate inadequate awareness regarding first aid algorithms for choking children and knowledge of the steps involved in FBAO treatment for an unresponsive paediatric patient [18].

The limited number and low quality of available data create a research gap, which needs further scientific investigation to improve evidence of healthcare providers' knowledge and competence in paediatric FBAO management. Medical students should receive training in first aid and possess knowledge on how to properly perform rescue manoeuvres for a choking child. Medical students may encounter choking cases in clinical or community settings. They may also need to educate parents, thereby equipping caregivers with the skills necessary to manage choking incidents. Basic prehospital emergency medicine skills are imperative for junior healthcare providers [19]. Although their competence in managing adult patients is generally extensive, there is limited information available concerning their proficiency in paediatric cases [20]. This raises the concern that adult-focused training may come at the expense of paediatric FBAO management.

Emergency management of choking is based on weak recommendations with very low certainty of scientific evidence [21]. Guidelines and algorithms regarding first aid for choking children differ across regions and organizations [22]. In infants (children aged 0–1 year) who have preserved consciousness but an ineffective cough, the guidelines are consistent throughout and recommend back blows as initial (first) and chest thrusts as secondary (second) rescue manoeuvres. Similarly, recommendations on when and how to implement cardiopulmonary resuscitation (CPR) are in accordance with each other. However, algorithms regarding first aid for choking children (age definitions varying by guideline, often ranging from 1 year to puberty) vary drastically (Table 1) [23–30].

Table 1. Comparison of algorithm differences in recommended manoeuvres and their sequence for managing foreign body airway obstruction in children older than 1 year old who have preserved consciousness but an ineffective cough.

	Back Blows	Chest Thrusts	Abdominal Thrusts
AHA [1]	not recommended	not recommended	only
ARC [2]	first	not recommended	second
CFAEG [3]	combine any two of the three options		
CRFAG [4]	not recommended	not recommended	only
ERC [5]	first	not recommended	second
RCSA [6]	second	not recommended	first
RLSS [7]/SJA [8]	first	not recommended	second

[1] AHA, American Heart Association; [2] ARC, American Red Cross; [3] CFAEG, Canadian First Aid Education Guidelines; [4] CRFAG, Canadian Resuscitation & First Aid Guidelines; [5] ERC, European Resuscitation Council; [6] RCSA, Resuscitation Council of Southern Africa; [7] RLSS, Royal Life Saving Society; [8] SJA, Saint John Ambulance.

These discrepancies may influence the effectiveness of FBAO management by both laypeople and healthcare providers. The lack of standardization could plausibly contribute to confusion among first aid providers, reducing their confidence and potentially affecting adherence to best practices. This, in turn, might result in variable applications of rescue manoeuvres and less predictable outcomes in time-sensitive emergencies. Further research is needed to assess the knowledge and competence of medical students in managing paediatric FBAO. This could improve future educational and training systems, help standardize divergent recommendations and guidelines, and ultimately, enhance outcomes for this vulnerable patient population.

With the aim of improving educational and training systems while simultaneously boosting the standardization of recommendations and guidelines and ultimately improving outcomes for vulnerable patient populations, future research should assess the knowledge and competence of medical students in managing paediatric FBAO. Gathered data can enrich scientific knowledge with previously unavailable information. Comparing distinct first aid education systems will reveal their advantages and disadvantages, enabling the identification of the most accessible and high-quality educational approach.

This study examines the knowledge and its sources of multinational medical students regarding first aid for paediatric FBAO. Given the absence of a universally validated and recommended emergency management algorithm based on scientific evidence, it is essential to assess medical students according to their specific, regional guidelines and training.

The detailed objectives of this study are as follows:

- Assess the preferred primary and secondary first aid rescue manoeuvres for children and infants with FBAO and determine their alignment with guidelines that influenced each participant's training program.
- Assess awareness of optimal positioning of the infant or child for these techniques.
- Evaluate how medical students manage a paediatric patient who has lost consciousness due to FBAO.
- Examine respondents' knowledge and attitudes regarding the use of anti-choking suction devices, the blind finger sweep manoeuvre, and the need for medical follow-ups for a child with restored airway patency.

2. Materials and Methods

2.1. Study Settings

A descriptive, cross-sectional study was conducted using an online survey developed by the authors. Data was collected from April 2024 to July 2024 from medical students in Canada, Libya, and Poland. The study was approved by the Bioethics Committee at the

Medical University of Lodz (number RNN/156/24/KE). The reporting of this study follows the STROBE (Strengthening the Reporting of Observational Studies in Epidemiology) statement (Supplementary Material S1).

2.2. Data Source

Data was collected through an online survey questionnaire (Supplementary File S1) created using the Microsoft Forms software (ver. 16.89.1 (24091630), Microsoft Corporation, Redmond, WA, USA) and distributed to participants via a QR code or direct link. To control for duplications of the responses, the survey platform was configured to allow only one response per email address.

The survey was designed to grant participants the greatest possible freedom to choose their course of action in order to examine, in the statistical analysis, the alignment of answers to the specific guidelines and not the correctness nor the order of the chosen rescue manoeuvres, as there is no globally unified algorithm of first aid management.

The first part of the questionnaire consisted of 4 sociodemographic questions and 4 questions devised to gather information about respondents' training process and experience. The second part of the questionnaire consisted of 4 open-ended questions: 2 focused on the first aid management of FBAO in an infant and 2 addressing FBAO in a 3-year-old child. After each question, medical students were asked to specify the positioning during the chosen lifesaving techniques. Respondents were also asked how they would manage a paediatric patient who has become unconscious due to FBAO. Further questions explored their views on the use of blind finger sweeps, the necessity of medical follow-ups after performing rescue manoeuvres, and their opinions on anti-choking suction devices.

Validation of the questionnaire was carried out using face and content validation techniques involving 24 participants from the target population. These respondents took part in structured interviews conducted by one of the researchers, during which they were asked to evaluate the questionnaire items for clarity, comprehensibility, consistency of interpretation, and neutrality. Adjustments were made based on feedback, using a five-point Likert-type evaluation scale.

This approach is consistent with established best practices for cognitive interviewing and pretesting, especially for open-ended and scenario-based instruments that are not intended for psychometric scaling. In such contexts, sample sizes ranging from 5 to 25 participants are considered sufficient for detecting major issues with question design and interpretation [31,32]. Therefore, the use of 24 pilot participants was deemed adequate for the aims of this stage of validation.

Full-scale psychometric validation (e.g., exploratory factor analysis or Cronbach's alpha) was not applicable given the structure and purpose of the instrument.

2.3. Participants

Medical students attending accredited institutions in Canada and Libya, as well as international students enrolled in the English Division at the Medical University of Łódź in Poland, were invited to participate to improve comprehension of the survey's language and cohesion within the studied groups. The choice of institution was dictated by previous cooperation, and the authors recognized the opportunity to conduct the study while maximizing multinational features to the extent that was available to them. Convenience sampling was used to recruit potential participants through recruitment posters displayed at educational facilities and emailed invitations to participate. Participation in the survey was voluntary and anonymous. An online information sheet explaining the purpose of the study and confidentiality of data was made available to all participants. Consent was implied by completing the survey. The inclusion criteria were willingness to participate in the study and a completed questionnaire. Although no a priori sample size calculation was performed due to the absence of a definable population frame, the adequacy of the sample was assessed through a post hoc sensitivity analysis. This study involved comparisons between 8 training council groups using categorical variables and chi-squared tests.

We chose 290 medical students to participate in the study through a convenience sampling method. However, the post hoc sensitivity analysis revealed that this sample size was sufficient to detect medium effect sizes (Cohen's w = 0.25) with 89.7% power at $\alpha = 0.05$ using chi-squared tests. This suggests that the collected sample was sufficiently large to identify statistically significant differences in the knowledge and adherence rates between groups.

2.4. Statistical Analysis

Statistical analysis was performed using the SPSS Statistics software (version 29.0.2.0), IBM Corp., Armonk, NY, USA) and RStudio version 4.3.3 (R Foundation for Statistical Computing, Vienna, Austria). Quantitative variables are presented using basic descriptive statistics: the arithmetic mean (x), standard deviation (SD), median (Me), minimum (Min), maximum (Max), interquartile range (IQR), and percentages (%). For comparisons where the expected frequencies were greater than five, distributions were analysed with the chi-squared test for independence. When the expectations were less than five, Fisher's exact test was chosen. Where the initial test indicates significance ($p < 0.05$ was considered significant, and $p < 0.01$ was considered highly significant), either the Benjamini–Hochberg False Discovery Rate post hoc test or the Bonferroni correction post hoc test was chosen to control for type-I errors, dependent on the dimension of the contingency table. Open-ended responses were consecutively reviewed manually with a qualitative content analysis and categorized thematically, and recurring patterns were summarized descriptively. This process was independently conducted by three authors, and the findings were then jointly reviewed by the entire group to ensure standardized and consistent conclusions.

3. Results

A total of 324 responses were received, and 13 responses were ineligible due to missing data and were discarded. Respondents were assigned to reference groups based on their responses to the question, "Have you received training on how to manage airway obstruction caused by foreign objects in children and infants?" Respondents, who self-reported no training ($n = 90$) were assigned to the untrained group and served as the control. Trained respondents were assigned to the guideline identification group ($n = 221$) according to self-reported data of which the training council's guidelines they had been taught and were subsequently categorized accordingly. Some respondents ($n = 21$) were excluded due to their inability to identify their training provider or with which guidelines/standards training was conducted (Figure 1).

A cohort of 290 medical students were included in the latter analysis. The mean age of the participants was 24.4 ± 3.9 (Me = 24; min = 18; max = 44). The majority of the participants were female (68.2%). A total of 98 (33.8%) respondents attended 9 Canadian universities (CA), 97 (33.4%) attended 2 Libyan universities (LY), and 95 (32.8%) attended 1 Polish university, with admission to programs in English language (PL-Eng). Despite attending medical institutions in only 3 countries, a total of 37 countries were reported by the participants when they were invited to identify their country of origin (Figure 2).

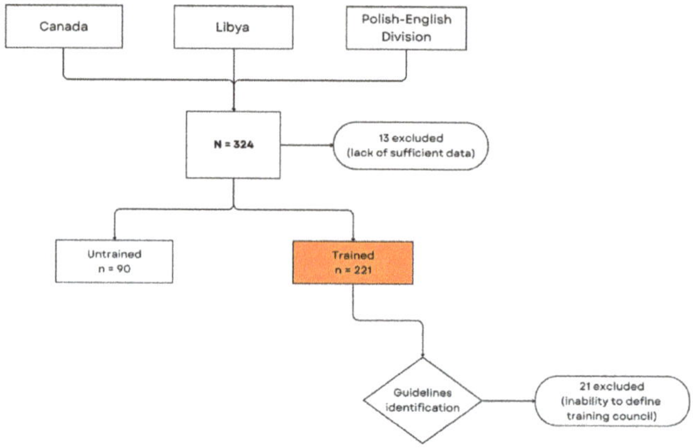

Figure 1. Flow chart of this paper methodology, process, and structure.

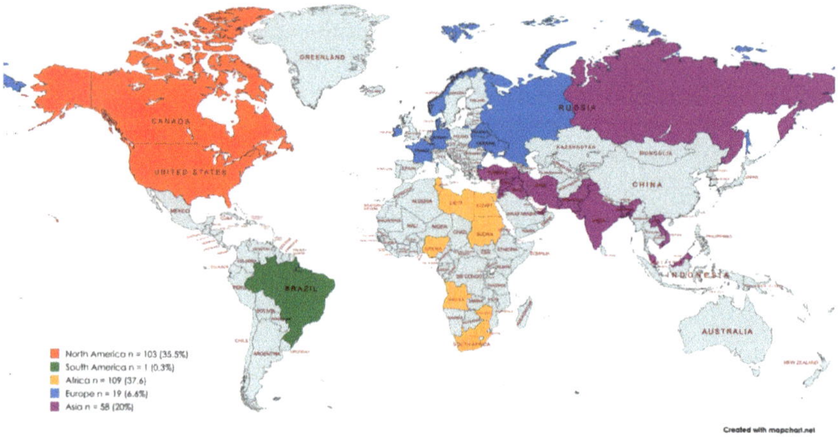

Figure 2. Diversity of participants' reported countries of origin, displayed by region.

Trained medical students were next divided into subgroups based on their answer to the question, "With which recommendation standards or resuscitation council did the training align?". From this procedure of guidelines identification, 7 new reference groups were formed, including the American Heart Association (AHA), American Red Cross (ARC), Canadian First Aid Education Guidelines (CFAEG), Canadian Resuscitation & First Aid Guidelines (CRFAG), the European Resuscitation Council (ERC), the Royal Life Saving Society (RLSS), Saint John Ambulance (SJA), and the Resuscitation Council of Southern Africa (RCSA) (Table 2).

Surveys of the participants were divided into 7 groups according to the guidelines on which they were trained, assessed by their answers to open-ended questions, and compared to the untrained group. This study evaluated the participants based on their first and second choice of rescue technique with the clinical scenario questions, "When you encounter an infant who is choking, showing signs of ineffective cough and maintaining consciousness, what should be your first manoeuvre to clear the airway?" (Infant—First Manoeuvre), and "When your first manoeuvre is unsuccessful and the infant is still choking, what should be your second manoeuvre to clear the airway?" (Infant—Second Manoeuvre). The questionaries also required respondents to specify how they would position the infant each time during the chosen rescue manoeuvre (Table 3).

The survey questions, "When you encounter a 3-year-old child who is choking, showing signs of ineffective cough and maintaining consciousness, what should be your first manoeuvre to clear the airway?" (Child—First Manoeuvre), and "When your first manoeuvre is unsuccessful, what should be your second manoeuvre to clear the airway?" (Child—Second Manoeuvre), assessed the medical students' knowledge of first aid for children using the same approach (Table 4).

Since the responses were open-ended, the terminology used was often not technical, and the answers had to be categorized. Groups were created accordingly, consisting of three mostly recommended rescue manoeuvres (abdominal thrusts, back blows, chest thrusts), with others categorized in one group (other) which comprised assessing the airway, a blind finger sweep of the oropharynx, encouragement of coughing, and changing the position of the infant for more comfort. As a result, both Tables 2 and 3 were shortened. The original, more precise tables are included in the Supplementary Materials (Supplementary File S3).

Then, a comparative analysis was carried out to evaluate the adherence of the above-described responses to the specific guidelines and assessed as to whether they were consistent with the training declared by the respondents (Figures 3 and 4).

Table 2. Participant characteristics.

N [1] = 290 n [2] (%)	**Canada**	**Libya**	**Polish–English Division**	**Total**
		Continent of Origin		
North America	98 (95.1)	0 (0)	5 (4.9)	103 (35.5)
Africa	0 (0)	89 (81.7)	20 (18.3)	109 (37.6)
Asia	0 (0)	6 (10.3)	52 (89.7)	58 (20)
Europe	0 (0)	2 (10.5)	17 (89.5)	19 (6.6)
South America	0 (0)	0 (0)	1 (100.0)	1 (0.3)
		Training Council		
AHA [3]	0 (0)	6 (40.0)	9 (60.0)	15 (4.8)
ARC [4]	1 (3.3)	29 (96.7)	0 (0)	30 (9.6)
CFAEG [5]	51 (100)	0 (0)	0 (0)	51 (16.4)
CRFAG [6]	23 (100)	0 (0)	0 (0)	23 (7.4)
ERC [7]	0 (0)	4 (6.1)	62 (93.9)	66 (21.2)
RLSS [8]/SJA [9]	13 (100)	0 (0)	0 (0)	13 (4.2)
RCSA [10]	0 (0)	0 (0)	2 (100)	2 (0.6)
Untrained	10 (11.1)	58 (64.4)	22 (24.4)	90 (28.9)

[1] N, population size; [2] n, sample size; [3] AHA, American Heart Association; [4] ARC, American Red Cross; [5] CFAEG, Canadian First Aid Education Guidelines; [6] CRFAG, Canadian Resuscitation & First Aid Guidelines; [7] ERC, European Resuscitation Council; [8] RCSA, Resuscitation Council of Southern Africa; [9] RLSS, Royal Life Saving Society; [10] SJA, Saint John Ambulance.

Table 3. Participant responses to clinical scenario questions by group (infant).

An Infant is Choking, Showing Signs of Ineffective Cough and Maintaining Consciousness. What Would be Your First Manoeuvre to Clear the Airway? (Infant—First Manoeuvre)									
Primary Intervention	AHA [1]	ARC [2]	CFAEG [3]	CRFAG [4]	ERC [5]	RCSA [6]	RLSS [7]/SJA [8]	Untrained	Total
n [9] (%)	15	30	51	23	66	2	13	90	290
Abdominal thrusts	1 (6.7)	0 (0)	0 (0)	0 (0)	4 (6.1)	0 (0)	0 (0)	7 (7.8)	12 (4.1)
Back blows	10 (66.7)	17 (56.7)	38 (74.5)	21 (91.3)	39 (59.1)	1 (50)	0 (0)	30 (33.3)	166 (57.2)
Chest thrusts	0 (0)	1 (3.3)	7 (13.7)	1 (4.3)	7 (10.6)	1 (50)	11 (84.6)	3 (3.3)	21 (7.2)
Other	4 (26.7)	12 (40)	6 (11.8)	1 (4.3)	16 (24.2)	0 (0)	2 (15.4)	50 (55.6)	91 (31.4)
Positioning during manoeuvre									
Lying flat on the ground	1 (6.7)	2 (6.7)	1 (2)	0 (0)	6 (9.1)	0 (0)	0 (0)	4 (4.4)	14 (4.8)
Lying flat on your lap	0 (0)	2 (6.7)	4 (7.8)	0 (0)	7 (10.6)	0 (0)	0 (0)	18 (20)	31 (10.7)
Lying on your lap with its head downwards	14 (93.3)	26 (86.7)	46 (90.2)	23 (100)	53 (80.3)	2 (100)	13 (100)	68 (75.6)	245 (84.5)
What would be your second manoeuvre to clear the airway if the first manoeuvre was unsuccessful and the patient's status is unchanged? (Infant—Second Manoeuvre)									
Abdominal thrusts	0 (0)	3 (10)	1 (2)	0 (0)	10 (15.2)	0 (0)	0 (0)	11 (12.2)	25 (8.6)
Back blows	2 (13.3)	7 (23.3)	16 (31.4)	2 (8.7)	9 (13.6)	2 (100)	2 (15.4)	14 (15.6)	54 (18.6)
Chest thrusts	10 (66.7)	17 (56.7)	32 (62.7)	21 (91.3)	32 (48.5)	0 (0)	11 (84.6)	19 (21.1)	142 (49)
Other	3 (20)	3 (10)	2 (3.9)	0 (0)	15 (22.7)	0 (0)	0 (0)	46 (51.1)	69 (23.8)
Positioning during manoeuvre									
Lying flat on the ground	3 (20)	5 (16.7)	0 (0)	0 (0)	7 (10.6)	0 (0)	0 (0)	18 (20)	33 (11.4)
Lying flat on your lap	9 (60)	9 (30)	16 (31.4)	2 (8.7)	31 (47)	0 (0)	2 (15.4)	23 (25.6)	92 (31.7)
Lying on your lap with its head downwards	3 (20)	16 (53.3)	35 (68.6)	21 (91.3)	28 (42.4)	2 (100)	11 (84.6)	49 (54.4)	165 (56.9)

[1] AHA, American Heart Association; [2] ARC, American Red Cross; [3] CFAEG, Canadian First Aid Education Guidelines; [4] CRFAG, Canadian Resuscitation & First Aid Guidelines; [5] ERC, European Resuscitation Council; [6] RCSA, Resuscitation Council of Southern Africa; [7] RLSS, Royal Life Saving Society; [8] SJA—Saint John Ambulance; [9] n, sample size.

Table 4. Participant responses to clinical scenario questions by group (child).

A 3-Year-Old Child is Choking, Showing Signs of Ineffective Cough and Maintaining Consciousness. What Would be Your First Manoeuvre to Clear the Airway? (Child—First Manoeuvre)									
Primary Intervention	AHA [1]	ARC [2]	CFAEG [3]	CRFAG [4]	ERC [5]	RCSA [6]	RLSS [7]/SJA [8]	Untrained	Total
n [9] (%)	15	30	51	23	66	2	13	90	290
Abdominal thrusts	4 (26.7)	4 (13.3)	13 (25.5)	8 (34.8)	13 (19.7)	0 (0)	5 (38.5)	21 (23.3)	68 (23.4)
Back blows	8 (53.3)	17 (56.7)	23 (45.1)	13 (56.5)	36 (54.5)	0 (0)	8 (61.5)	25 (27.8)	130 (44.8)
Chest thrusts	0 (0)	0 (0)	0 (0)	0 (0)	1 (1.5)	0 (0)	0 (0)	0 (0)	1 (0.3)
Other	3 (20)	9 (30)	15 (29.4)	2 (8.7)	17 (24.3)	2 (100)	0 (0)	44 (48.9)	91 (31.5)
Positioning during manoeuvre									
	0 (0)	2 (6.7)	1 (2)	0 (0)	6 (9.1)	0 (0)	0 (0)	4 (4.4)	14 (4.8)
Sitting upright	1 (6.7)	1 (3.3)	0 (0)	0 (0)	4 (6.1)	0 (0)	0 (0)	8 (8.9)	14 (4.8)
Sitting with a forward lean	4 (26.7)	4 (13.3)	1 (2)	0 (0)	8 (12.1)	0 (0)	1 (7.7)	16 (17.8)	34 (11.7)
Standing upright	3 (20)	3 (10)	9 (17.6)	6 (26.1)	4 (6.1)	0 (0)	4 (30.8)	16 (17.8)	45 (15.5)
Standing upright with a forward lean	7 (46.7)	22 (73.3)	41 (80.4)	17 (73.9)	50 (75.8)	2 (100)	8 (61.5)	50 (55.6)	197 (67.9)
What would be your second manoeuvre to clear the airway if the first manoeuvre was unsuccessful and the patient's status is unchanged? (Child—Second Manoeuvre)									
Abdominal thrusts	8 (53.3)	15 (50)	25 (49)	15 (65.3)	34 (51.5)	0 (0)	6 (46.1)	23 (25.5)	126 (43.4)
Back blows	1 (6.7)	4 (13.3)	18 (35.3)	7 (30.4)	9 (13.6)	2 (100)	5 (38.5)	9 (10)	55 (19.0)
Chest thrusts	1 (6.7)	3 (10)	7 (13.7)	1 (4.3)	6 (9.1)	0 (0)	2 (15.4)	3 (3.3)	23 (7.9)
Other	5 (33.3)	8 (26.7)	1 (2)	0 (0)	17 (25.8)	0 (0)	0 (0)	55 (61)	86 (29.7)
Positioning during manoeuvre									
Sitting upright	0 (0)	1 (3.3)	0 (0)	0 (0)	0 (0)	0 (0)	1 (7.7)	7 (7.8)	9 (3.1)
Sitting with a forward lean	0 (0)	5 (16.7)	1 (2)	0 (0)	8 (12.1)	0 (0)	0 (0)	24 (26.7)	38 (13.1)
Standing upright	3 (20)	7 (23.3)	16 (31.4)	9 (39.1)	24 (36.4)	0 (0)	3 (23.1)	16 (17.8)	78 (26.9)
Standing upright with a forward lean	12 (80)	17 (56.7)	34 (66.7)	14 (60.9)	34 (51.5)	2 (100)	9 (69.2)	43 (47.8)	165 (56.9)

[1] AHA, American Heart Association; [2] ARC, American Red Cross; [3] CFAEG, Canadian First Aid Education Guidelines; [4] CRFAG, Canadian Resuscitation & First Aid Guidelines; [5] ERC, European Resuscitation Council; [6] RCSA, Resuscitation Council of Southern Africa; [7] RLSS, Royal Life Saving Society; [8] SJA—Saint John Ambulance; [9] n, sample size.

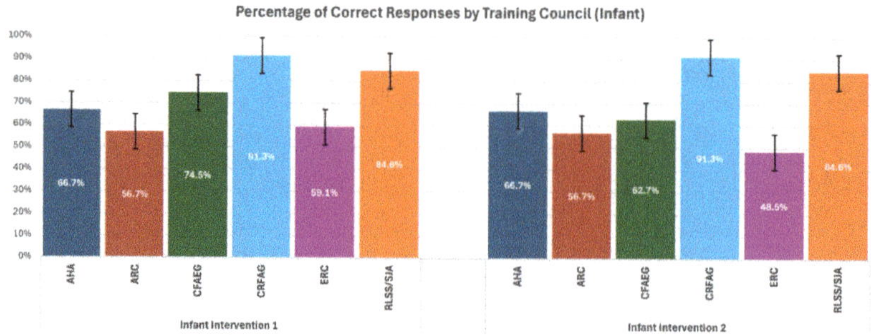

Figure 3. Response adherence by training council for infant interventions.

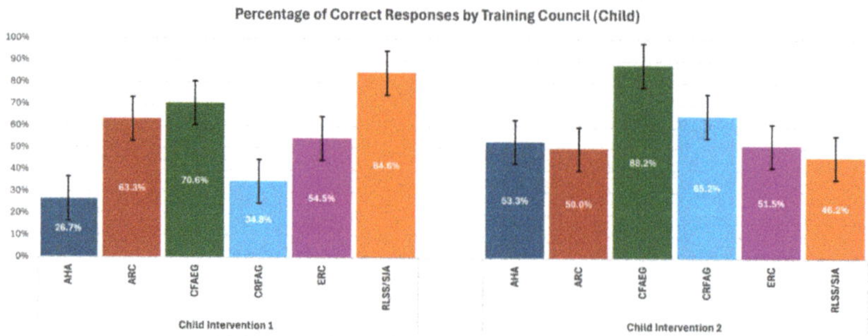

Figure 4. Response adherence by training council for child interventions.

The data from four different scenarios was analysed through Fisher's exact test, which is appropriate for small sample sizes and contingency tables with expected frequencies less than 5. The results indicate the following:

- Infant—First Manoeuvre:

Fisher's exact test resulted in a p-value of 0.007659, indicating that there are statistically significant differences among the different training councils in the adherence to the first rescue manoeuvre in a choking infant scenario. This suggests that some guidelines may perform better than others in this clinical situation. However, the post hoc analysis showed no significant differences between the specific pairs of groups after adjusting for multiple comparisons (FDR correction), implying that while there is an overall significant effect, the differences between any individual training council were not significant at the 95% confidence level.

- Infant—Second Manoeuvre:

For the second rescue manoeuvre for helping a choking infant scenario, the p-value of 0.001414 suggests a significant effect, indicating differences in adherence to the algorithm for infants between the different training councils. Post hoc testing revealed that there is a statistically significant difference between ERC and CRFAG councils ($p = 0.00794$), showing that guidelines from different councils may lead to notable variations in the application of the algorithm.

- Child—First Manoeuvre:

For the first rescue manoeuvre for a conscious child who is choking, the p-value of 0.001192 indicates differences in the adherence rates. Post hoc analyses highlighted significant pairwise differences between the following:

- AHA vs. CFAEG (adjusted $p = 0.0304$);
- AHA vs. RLSS/SJA (adjusted $p = 0.0304$);
- CFAEG vs. CRFAG (adjusted $p = 0.0304$);
- CRFAG vs. RLSS/SJA (adjusted $p = 0.0304$).

These findings suggest that the respondents trained by opposed training councils differ in their choice of first rescue manoeuvre for choking children. In these pairs, CFAEG, RLSS/SJA, CFAEG, and RLSS/SJA, respectively, performed better.

- Child—Second Manoeuvre:

Fisher's exact test yielded a p-value of 0.0001921, indicating a high statistical difference in adherence between the councils. The FDR post hoc analysis revealed significant differences between the following:

- AHA vs. CFAEG (adjusted $p = 0.034$);
- ARC vs. CFAEG (adjusted $p = 0.00432$);
- CFAEG vs. ERC (adjusted $p = 0.000479$);
- CFAEG vs. RLSS/SJA (adjusted $p = 0.0182$).

This indicates that some respondents have a stronger adherence to the algorithm for second rescue manoeuvre for choking children than others, with CFAEG performing notably better in several pairwise comparisons.

Figure 5 was created to better visualize the overall adherence percentage for each training council, combining the results from all four scenarios.

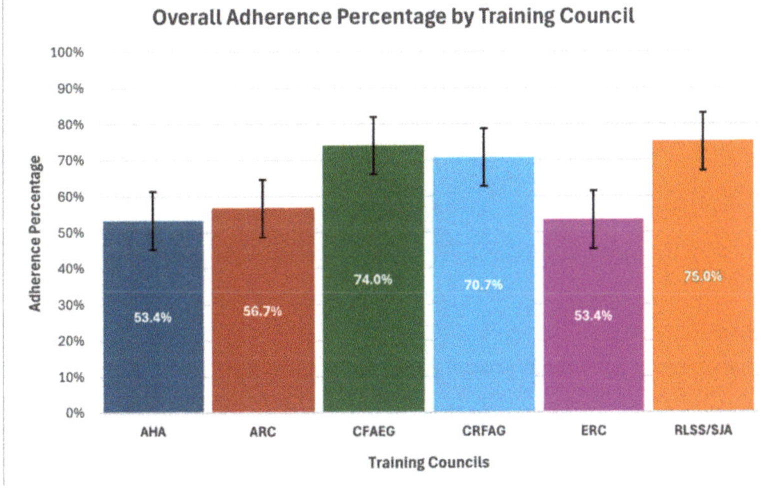

Figure 5. Overall adherence percentage by training council.

Additionally, the respondents were also asked, "What steps would you take if an infant or a child who is choking loses consciousness and stops to breathe—explain the sequence of actions that should be followed", in order to examine their ability to recognize cardiac arrest caused by FBAO and implement CPR (Table 5).

Furthermore, the problems of anti-choking suction devices (ACSDs), medical follow-ups, and blind finger sweeping were explored. Participants were asked the questions, "Is it recommended to utilize anti-choking suction devices in the first aid of a choking child?", "If the foreign body airway obstruction is relieved, is it necessary to routinely seek urgent medical follow-up from a professional?", and "Would you attempt a blind finger sweep manoeuvre in this scenario to attempt to clear the obstruction by using your finger to remove not visible object?" (Table 6).

Table 5. Participant responses to clinical questions by group (CPR).

Primary Intervention	AHA [1]	ARC [2]	CFAEG [3]	CRFAG [4]	ERC [5]	RCSA [6]	RLSS [7]/SJA [8]	Untrained	Total
n [9] (%)	15	30	51	23	66	2	13	90	290
What steps would you take if an infant or a child is choking, loses consciousness, and stops breathing									
Request help/EMS [10]	7 (46.7)	8 (26.7)	20 (39.2)	15 (65.2)	26 (39.4)	0 (0)	10 (79.6)	17 (18.9)	103 (35.5)
CPR [11]	10 (66.7)	21 (70)	39 (76.5)	23 (100)	46 (69.7)	2 (100)	13 (100)	32 (35.6)	186 (64.1)
Chest thrusts or back blows	1 (6.7)	5 (16.7)	9 (17.6)	0 (0)	10 (15.2)	0 (0)	0 (0)	8 (8.9)	33 (11.4)
Unsure	1 (6.7)	5 (16.7)	3 (5.9)	0 (0)	4 (6.1)	0 (0)	0 (0)	36 (40)	49 (16.9)

[1] AHA, American Heart Association; [2] ARC, American Red Cross; [3] CFAEG, Canadian First Aid Education Guidelines; [4] CRFAG, Canadian Resuscitation & First Aid Guidelines; [5] ERC, European Resuscitation Council; [6] RCSA, Resuscitation Council of Southern Africa; [7] RLSS, Royal Life Saving Society; [8] SJA, Saint John Ambulance; [9] n, population; [10] EMS, Emergency Medical Services; [11] CPR, Cardiopulmonary Resuscitation.

Table 6. Participant responses to clinical questions by group (ACSDs, medical follow-ups, and blind finger sweeping).

Primary Intervention	AHA [1]	ARC [2]	CFAEG [3]	CRFAG [4]	ERC [5]	RCSA [6]	RLSS [7]/SJA [8]	Untrained	Total
n [9] (%)	15	30	51	23	66	2	13	90	290
Is it recommended to utilize anti-choking suction devices in the first aid of a choking child?									
Yes	3 (20)	3 (10)	3 (5.9)	0 (0)	13 (19.7)	2 (100)	0 (0)	24 (26.7)	48 (16.6)
No	2 (13.4)	15 (50)	18 (35.3)	15 (65.2)	13 (19.7)	0 (0)	8 (61.5)	10 (11.1)	81 (27.9)
Unsure	10 (66.7)	12 (40)	30 (58.8)	8 (34.8)	40 (60.6)	0 (0)	5 (38.5)	56 (62.2)	161 (55.5)
If the foreign body airway obstruction is relieved, is it necessary to routinely seek urgent medical follow-up?									
Yes	6 (40)	11 (36.7)	47 (92.2)	19 (82.6)	46 (70.7)	2 (100)	10 (76.9)	55 (61.1)	196 (67.6)
No	6 (40)	8 (26.7)	2 (3.9)	2 (8.7)	11 (16.7)	0 (0)	1 (7.7)	12 (13.3)	42 (14.5)
Unsure	3 (20)	11 (36.7)	2 (3.9)	2 (8.7)	9 (13.6)	0	2 (15.4)	23 (25.6)	52 (17.9)
Would you perform a blind finger sweep to remove an unseen obstruction?									
Yes	3 (20)	1 (3.3)	6 (11.8)	0 (0)	15 (22.7)	2 (100)	0 (0)	15 (16.7)	42 (14.5)
No	7 (46.7)	23 (76.7)	38 (74.5)	22 (95.7)	37 (56.1)	0 (0)	12 (92.3)	39 (43.3)	178 (61.4)
Unsure	5 (33.4)	6 (20)	7 (13.7)	1 (4.3)	14 (21.2)	0 (0)	1 (7.7)	36 (40)	70 (24.1)

[1] AHA, American Heart Association; [2] ARC, American Red Cross; [3] CFAEG, Canadian First Aid Education Guidelines; [4] CRFAG, Canadian Resuscitation & First Aid Guidelines; [5] ERC, European Resuscitation Council; [6] RCSA, Resuscitation Council of Southern Africa; [7] RLSS, Royal Life Saving Society; [8] SJA, Saint John Ambulance; [9] n, population.

4. Discussion

This study reveals substantial variability in knowledge retention across training councils, with RLSS/SJA consistently outperforming others. However, the small sample size in this group makes these findings less generalizable. CFAEG achieved the highest adherence rates on average in most scenarios. This highlights the efficacy of their training approach, likely attributed to detailed, simulation-based curricula that reinforce long-term retention. In contrast, AHA, while globally prominent, showed relatively poor adherence in Child—First Manoeuvre, indicating potential gaps in their teaching methodologies for paediatric choking scenarios. Similarly, ERC displayed moderate but inconsistent results for Infant—Second Manoeuvre. CRFAG performed exceptionally well in infant scenarios yet had lower success rates with first rescue manoeuvres for child choking. This disparity may reflect differences in emphasis during training or the complexity of certain algorithms.

In clinical scenario questions regarding helping a choking infant and choosing first rescue manoeuvres, we found significant differences among the councils; this suggests that some guidelines may be more effective in training. Although no specific pairwise differences were significant in the post hoc analysis, this still indicates that the chosen guidelines significantly influence performance. For questions regarding the choice of the second rescue manoeuvre, we found significant differences between CRFAG and ERC groups; this implies that some councils might have more effective methods for teaching. It would be beneficial to explore these differences further to refine training protocols globally. Furthermore, clinical scenario questions regarding helping a choking child and choosing first rescue manoeuvres found significant findings that suggest certain councils (such as CFAEG) may provide superior training, which leads to better adherence to choking management procedures. Sharing best practices among councils could help improve global outcomes. In questions where medical students had to choose a second rescue manoeuvre, very significant differences between councils where found, which emphasizes the need for standardized training materials that ensure higher consistency in the application of emergency procedures. CFAEG and CRFAG, in particular, performed well and might serve as a model for improving other councils' protocols.

In all of the aforementioned clinical scenario questions, an additional assessment of positioning in which chosen rescue manoeuvres would be performed was carried out. This consideration has never been studied before, and no scientific evidence exist; however, it seems plausible that positioning may have some impact on the effectiveness and safety of the rescue manoeuvre, due to the influence of gravity on the foreign body and a more convenient anatomical positioning of the airway. This can potentially occur when a victim is placed in a position with a forward lean, and their head is pointed downwards [33]. Additional aspects of ergonomics exist, e.g., placing the child on the rescuer's lap or forearm [34,35]. In Infant—First Manoeuvre, a significant portion of the respondents understood this concept. However, in Infant—Second Manoeuvre, some difficulties occurred, most likely caused by doubts regarding the rescue manoeuvres themselves. In Child—First Manoeuvre and Child—Second Manoeuvre, the respondents were more in agreement that the victim should be standing with a forward lean.

The use of Fisher's exact test was appropriate given the small sample sizes and non-normal distributions. The significant p-values suggest strong evidence that different councils do indeed lead to different outcomes in choking scenario adherence. However, the pairwise comparisons (post hoc tests) showed that only certain groups had significant differences, which suggests that while there is a general trend, the differences are not uniform across all comparisons.

In the question about a child who experienced a sudden cardiac arrest after a choking episode, CPR was attempted by 64.1% of the respondents, which is a worrying result. The best performance was achieved by the CRFAG group and RLS/SJA and RCSA, although the latter were significantly limited in the number of participants. The remaining groups achieved a similar result, not distinguishing themselves significantly from each other. A small group noted that they would call for help from professionals; CRFAG and RLS/SJA stood out, with an average response of 65.2% and 79.6%, respectively. The remaining respondents would implement chest thrusts or back blows or did not know what to do in this situation, or their answers were considered incorrect, because they are not recommended in any guidelines. The importance of CPR in unresponsive patients after a choking incident has been established and supported by research repeatedly. Choking followed by severe brain tissue hypoxia causes cardiac arrest with extremely poor prognosis, especially when patients are not immediately resuscitated by witnesses through first aid [27,36].

Additional aspects of first aid in FBAO, such as ACSDs, medical follow-ups, and blind finger sweeping, were explored in order to select the group of respondents with the best level of understanding of these subsidiary issues. The guidelines gathered in this study are consistent in their recommendations regarding the above aspects. Firstly, the utilization of ACSDs gave a lot of doubts to the medical students, which may be due to the fact that many guidelines do not emphasize this topic enough [23–30]. They are not recommended due to lack of evidence, but there is a growing trend of describing and studying them in the scientific literature [22,37,38]. The respondents from CRFAG, RLSS/SJA, and ARC had the highest percentage of correct answers, while the rest were mostly incorrect or unsure. Secondly, the position on medical follow-ups after the application of rescue manoeuvres is also well unified across the guidelines. As FBAO can cause airway trauma and external forces applied during assistance procedures may also result in injuries, it is recommended to consult a physician after such an event. However, not all respondents had this information well assimilated, as less than half of the AHA and ARC groups chose not to seek a medical follow-up, performing worse than the untrained individuals. Thirdly, the knowledge and attitude toward blind finger sweeping the oropharynx was assessed to determine the quality of the guidelines learned, as all training councils do not support it. Again, the greatest awareness of the problem was shown by the respondents trained by CRFAG and RLSS/SJA. The worst performers were the students from the AHA and ERC groups, almost at the level of the untrained students. The RCSA group was willing to use this procedure, but it must be remembered that this was a very small and unrepresentative group.

This study's findings also highlight the importance of training, as the untrained respondents provided responses that were significantly poorer, nearly double that of the trained respondents. The majority of the untrained respondents answered, "I am not sure". This seems to be consistent with existing evidence [39–41]. The sole existence of medical students that are not trained in basic first aid is very worrying. Three countries partook in the study, and in each, first aid is embedded and taught across the academic curriculum or required as a program prerequisite for entry. However, the volunteers who took part in the study came from different nations and individual backgrounds, meaning that their origins further remain unknown. This prompts a reflection of the educational systems of not only medical students but also of children and youth with regard to teaching and learning first aid with the aim of improving patient survival of FBAO.

This study is among the first to map medical student knowledge of paediatric FBAO interventions against specific training council guidelines across multiple countries. By identifying clear differences in adherence tied to curricular exposure, the findings provide empirical support for harmonizing guideline content in medical education. Rather than broadly identifying knowledge gaps, this study points to specific areas, such as confusion around back blows versus abdominal thrusts, where targeted educational improvements could improve consistency and safety in paediatric emergency response.

4.1. Proposal of Practical Implications

- Focus on Standardization: Given the variability in adherence rates, harmonizing training protocols across international councils could bridge knowledge gaps and improve outcomes globally.
- Enhanced Training Techniques: The superior performance of CFAEG and CRFAG highlights the importance of simulation-based training, which may serve as a model for other organizations.
- Targeted Interventions for Underperforming Regions: Customizing training to the local context, as well as increasing accessibility to high-quality materials, could help underperforming councils improve.
- Periodic Assessments: Longitudinal studies to assess knowledge retention over time and its correlation with real-world competence should be prioritized.

4.2. Recommendations for Future Research

There are significant differences in adherence to guideline-recommended manoeuvres, with some councils demonstrating superior outcomes. Future research should focus on follow-up studies analysing the instructional methods employed by these councils and how they differ from others. Research should focus on exploring the reasons that could not be examined in this study, such as a deeper analysis of training methods (e.g., simulation-based or highly structured pedagogical models), cultural differences in training acceptance, and the impact of refresher courses or long-term retention. It may also be valuable to investigate how training delivery (e.g., in person vs. online) impacts adherence to guidelines, as this could be another contributing factor to the observed differences.

5. Limitations

This study has several limitations. Firstly, the problem of guideline identification arose during the statistical analysis and assigning respondents to the groups, as some of them could not identify their training council. As a result, a number of the questionnaires had to be excluded. This could be corrected in future studies by focusing their scope to a specific group of individuals who are aware of their training or where their training is known. Secondly, the questionnaires did not examine the year or level of education of the respondents, which could potentially have some effects on their knowledge; however, it is unlikely that this would have any influence on their adherence to guidelines or training councils. On the other hand, further examination of knowledge retention by assessing factors such as the year of medical training could enhance the findings. Additionally, other potential confounding factors were not extensively examined. These include institutional differences across universities, potential differences in education curriculum and level, graduating from another medical speciality in the past, and different course methodologies. Thirdly, this study did not assess encouraging coughing in conscious children with an effective cough, as this action is not an actual rescue manoeuvre and is typically straightforward and universally recommended, being less subject to variation in medical education. Fourthly, the data was gathered from three countries, which gives some collective value to the findings. Nevertheless, not all of it should be applied globally, as the limited geographic and institutional distribution may restrict the results from broader applications. Fifthly, the responses were based on self-assessments and participant recall, which may have been influenced by the social desirability bias or may be inaccurate due to limitations in memory. These factors, along with the exploratory nature of preferred body positioning during rescue manoeuvres and attitudes toward anti-choking suction devices, should prompt cautious interpretation due to the lack of practical validation and differences in the groups' sample sizes.

6. Conclusions

This study identified observable differences in knowledge and adherence to paediatric choking rescue guidelines among medical students trained under different international standards. Certain educational institutions manage to produce better results in terms of adherence to choking intervention guidelines regarding primary and secondary first aid rescue manoeuvres as well as cardiopulmonary resuscitation for children and infants. These descriptive findings may reflect underlying variations in the structure and content of training curricula. Although no multivariate analysis was performed, the results suggest that curricular harmonization might be a useful direction to explore in future studies aiming to improve consistency and preparedness in paediatric emergency response. Additional differences were discovered in the degree of awareness regarding such problems like body positioning, anti-choking suction devices, the blind finger sweep manoeuvre, and the need for medical follow-ups for a child with restored airway patency. Further research is needed to understand the factors that lead to such differences in training program outcomes and how they can be minimized to improve global choking management quality.

Supplementary Materials: The following supporting information can be downloaded at: https://www.mdpi.com/article/10.3390/healthcare13121441/s1, File S1: STROBE checklist; File S2: Online survey questionnaire; File S3: Table S1: Participant responses to clinical scenario questions by group (infant); Table S2: Participant responses to clinical scenario questions by group (child).

Author Contributions: Conceptualization, J.R.B. and F.J.; methodology, F.J.; software, F.J.; validation, J.R.B. and F.J.; formal analysis, J.R.B., R.H. and F.J.; investigation, J.R.B., R.H. and F.J.; resources, J.R.B., R.H. and F.J.; data curation, J.R.B., R.H. and F.J.; writing—original draft preparation, J.R.B., R.H. and F.J.; writing—review and editing, J.R.B., R.H., F.J., K.N. and D.T.; visualization, F.J.; supervision, F.J., K.N. and D.T. All authors have read and agreed to the published version of the manuscript.

Funding: This research received no external funding.

Institutional Review Board Statement: The study was conducted in accordance with the Declaration of Helsinki and approved by the Bioethics Committee of the Medical University of Lodz (number RNN/156/24/KE).

Informed Consent Statement: Not applicable.

Data Availability Statement: The data presented in this study is available on reasonable request from the corresponding author due to restrictions resulting from the policy of the Bioethics Committee.

Acknowledgments: We would like to express our deep appreciation for the assistance of Ibrahim El-Gehani in data collection from Libya and Connor J. O'Keefe for statistical consultation from Canada.

Conflicts of Interest: F.J. is the founder, medical consultant, and co-constructor of the "ECO CPR" project, financed by the programme "Innovation Incubator 4.0" as part of the non-competitive project entitled "Support for the management of scientific research and commercialization of the results of R&D works in scientific units and enterprises" under the Intelligent Development Operational Program 2014–2020 (Measure 4.4). There are no other conflicts of interest or financial relationships with manufacturers or products to declare. F.J. is the Guest Editor of the Special Issue "A Needle in a Haystack: Looking for Gaps in Treatment and Education in Emergency Medicine" and declares a potential conflict of interest due to their role as a co-supervisor of the doctoral candidate—J.R.B.—who co-authored the submitted manuscript. The editorial and peer review process was managed independently without any involvement of the Guest Editor in the decision-making or review procedures. D.T. is the President of the Polish Society for Emergency Medicine (2023–2027). J.R.B., R.H., and K.N. have no conflicts of interest to declare.

References

1. Dodson, H.; Cook, J. *Foreign Body Airway Obstruction*; StatPearls Publishing [Internet]: Treasure Island, FL, USA, 2023.
2. White, J.J.; Cambron, J.D.; Gottlieb, M.; Long, B. Evaluation and Management of Airway Foreign Bodies in the Emergency Department Setting. *J. Emerg. Med.* **2023**, *64*, 145–155. [CrossRef] [PubMed]
3. Fano, C.; Lorenzoni, G.; Azzolina, D.; Giuliani, A.; French, M.; Campagna, S.; Berchialla, P.; Gregori, D. Perception of Choking Injury Risk Among Healthcare Students. *J. Community Health* **2019**, *44*, 974–981. [CrossRef] [PubMed]
4. Foltran, F.; Ballali, S.; Rodriguez, H.; Sebastian van As, A.B.; Passali, D.; Gulati, A.; Gregori, D. Inhaled foreign bodies in children: A global perspective on their epidemiological, clinical, and preventive aspects. *Pediatr. Pulmonol.* **2013**, *48*, 344–351. [CrossRef] [PubMed]
5. Erikci, V.S. Airway Foreign Bodies in Children: A Review Article. *J. Clin. Res. Rep.* **2022**, *11*, 1–4. [CrossRef]
6. Landoni, G.; Morselli, F.; Silvetti, S.; Frontera, A.; Zangrillo, A.; Collaborators. Pizza in adults and grape in children are the most frequent causes of foreign body airway obstruction in Italy. A national media-based survey. *Resuscitation* **2020**, *149*, 141–142. [CrossRef]
7. Igarashi, Y.; Suzuki, K.; Norii, T.; Motomura, T.; Yoshino, Y.; Kitagoya, Y.; Ogawa, S.; Yokobori, S.; Yokota, H. Do Video Calls Improve Dispatcher-Assisted First Aid for Infants with Foreign Body Airway Obstruction? A Randomized Controlled Trial/Simulation Study. *J. Nippon Med. Sch.* **2022**, *89*, 526–532. [CrossRef]
8. Lott, C.; Truhlář, A.; Alfonzo, A.; Barelli, A.; González-Salvado, V.; Hinkelbein, J.; Nolan, J.P.; Paal, P.; Perkins, G.D.; Thies, K.C.; et al. European Resuscitation Council Guidelines 2021: Cardiac arrest in special circumstances. *Resuscitation* **2021**, *161*, 152–219. [CrossRef]

9. Ngamsanga, S.; Vathanophas, V.; Ungkanont, K.; Tanphaichitr, A.; Wannarong, T. Pediatric respiratory tract foreign bodies in children: A systematic review. *Auris Nasus Larynx* **2023**, *50*, 607–613. [CrossRef]
10. Tse, E.; Plakitsi, K.; Voulgaris, S.; Alexiou, G.A. ChokeSafe: Empowering Children with Life-Saving Choking-Management Skills. *Children* **2024**, *11*, 299. [CrossRef]
11. León-Guereño, P.; Cid-Aldama, L.; Galindo-Domínguez, H.; Amezua-Urrutia, A. Effectiveness of an Intervention to Enhance First Aid Knowledge among Early Childhood Education Students: A Pilot Study. *Children* **2023**, *10*, 1252. [CrossRef]
12. Wani, J.I.; Almushayt, N.O.; Abbag, W.F.; Buhran, L.A.; Nadeem, M. Pediatric first aid, trauma knowledge, and attitude among parents and general population in Aseer region, Southern Saudi Arabia. *SAGE Open Med.* **2022**, *14*, 10. [CrossRef] [PubMed]
13. Ranjous, Y.; Al Balkhi, A.; Alnader, I.; Rkab, M.; Ataya, J.; Abouharb, R. Knowledge and misconceptions of choking and first-aid procedures among Syrian adults: A cross-sectional study. *SAGE Open Med.* **2024**, *8*, 12. [CrossRef] [PubMed]
14. Habeeb, K.A.; Alarfaj, G. Saudi parents awareness regarding burn, choking, and drowning first aid in children. *J. Fam. Med. Prim. Care* **2020**, *9*, 1370–1375. [CrossRef]
15. Maalim, I.A.; Jiru, T.; Wubetie, A.A. Assessment of knowledge, attitude and practice on first aid management of choking and associated factors among kindergarten teachers in Addis Ababa governmental schools, Addis Ababa, Ethiopia. A cross-sectional institution-based study. *PLoS ONE* **2021**, *16*, e0255331. [CrossRef]
16. Hosapatna, M.; Bhat, N.; Belle, J.; Priyadarshini, S.; Ankolekar, V.H. Knowledge and Training of Primary School Teachers in First Aid—A Questionnaire Based Study. *Kurume Med. J.* **2021**, *66*, 101–106. [CrossRef] [PubMed]
17. Meerkov, M.S.; Fischer, J.B.; Saba, T.G. A simulation procedure curriculum to increase pediatric resident exposure to procedures rarely performed in clinical practice. *Med. Educ. Online* **2019**, *24*, 1611305. [CrossRef]
18. Butler, M.W.; Adefuye, A.O. Assessing the knowledge of emergency medical care personnel in the Free State, South Africa, on aspects of paediatric pre-hospital emergency care. *Pan Afr. Med. J.* **2019**, *32*, 98.
19. Antrum, J.H.; Ho, J.K. Prehospital emergency care: Why training should be compulsory for medical undergraduates. *Emerg. Med. J.* **2015**, *32*, 171–172. [CrossRef]
20. Sturny, L.; Regard, S.; Larribau, R.; Niquille, M.; Savoldelli, G.L.; Sarasin, F.; Schiffer, E.; Suppan, L. Differences in Basic Life Support Knowledge Between Junior Medical Students and Lay People: Web-Based Questionnaire Study. *J. Med. Internet Res.* **2021**, *23*, e25125. [CrossRef]
21. Berg, K.M.; Bray, J.E.; Ng, K.C.; Liley, H.G.; Greif, R.; Carlson, J.N.; Morley, P.T.; Drennan, I.R.; Smyth, M.; Scholefield, B.R.; et al. 2023 International Consensus on Cardiopulmonary Resuscitation and Emergency Cardiovascular Care Science With Treatment Recommendations: Summary From the Basic Life Support; Advanced Life Support; Pediatric Life Support; Neonatal Life Support; Education, Implementation, and Teams; and First Aid Task Forces. *Circulation* **2023**, *148*, 187–280. [CrossRef]
22. Bieliński, J.R.; Huntley, R.; Dunne, C.L.; Timler, D.; Nadolny, K.; Jaskiewicz, F. Do We Actually Help Choking Children? The Quality of Evidence on the Effectiveness and Safety of First Aid Rescue Manoeuvres: A Narrative Review. *Medicina* **2024**, *60*, 1827. [CrossRef]
23. Topjian, A.A.; Raymond, T.T.; Atkins, D.; Chan, M.; Duff, J.P.; Joyner, B.L., Jr.; Lasa, J.J.; Lavonas, E.J.; Levy, A.; Mahgoub, M.; et al. Pediatric Basic and Advanced Life Support Collaborators. Part 4: Pediatric Basic and Advanced Life Support: 2020 AmericanHeart Association Guidelines for Cardiopulmonary Resuscitation and Emergency Cardiovascular Care. *Circulation* **2020**, *20*, 469–523.
24. American Red Cross. Adult/Child Choking. Available online: https://www.redcross.org/take-a-class/resources/learn-first-aid/adult-child-choking (accessed on 1 January 2025).
25. Canadian First Aid Education Guidelines. The Canadian Red Cross Society. 2020. Available online: https://www.redcross.ca/training-and-certification/first-aid-tips-and-resources/canadian-first-aid-education-guidelines (accessed on 1 January 2025).
26. Canadian Resuscitation; First Aid Guidelines. Heart & Stroke Foundation of Canada. 2020. Available online: https://cpr.heartandstroke.ca/s/article/Guidelines (accessed on 1 January 2025).
27. Van de Voorde, P.; Turner, N.M.; Djakow, J.; de Lucas, N.; Martinez-Mejias, A.; Biarent, D.; Bingham, R.; Brissaud, O.; Hoffmann, F.; Johannesdottir, G.B.; et al. European Resuscitation Council Guidelines 2021: Paediatric Life Support. *Resuscitation* **2021**, *61*, 327–387. [CrossRef]
28. The Resuscitation Council of Southern Africa. Choking. Available online: https://resus.co.za/Documents/Algorithms/RESUS%20CHOKING%20ALGORITHM.pdf (accessed on 1 January 2025).
29. Royal Life Saving Society Canada. *Canadian First Aid Manual*, 8th ed.; Royal Life Saving Society Canada, Alberta & Northwest Territories Branch and Ontario Branch: Toronto, ON, Canada, 2021.
30. St John Ambulance. First Aid Reference Guide. St. John Ambulance Canada. 2024 Feb. Available online: https://sja.ca/sites/default/files/2024-03/FARG_February%202024_EN_0.pdf (accessed on 1 January 2025).
31. Willis, G.B. *Cognitive Interviewing: A Tool for Improving Questionnaire Design*; Sage Publications: Thousand Oaks, CA, USA, 2005.
32. Artino, A.R.; La Rochelle, J.S.; Dezee, K.J.; Gehlbach, H. Developing questionnaires for educational research: AMEE Guide No. 87. *Med. Teach.* **2014**, *36*, 463–474. [CrossRef] [PubMed]

33. Luczak, A. Effect of body position on relieve of foreign body from the airway. *AIMS Public Health* **2019**, *6*, 154–159. [CrossRef]
34. Gesicki, A.; Longmore, S. Time to Reconsider the Straddle-Arm Technique: Providing Care for the Conscious Infant who is Choking. *Int. J. First Aid Educ.* **2019**, *2*, 67. [CrossRef]
35. Gesicki, A.; Chan, A. An Alternative to the Straddle-Arm Technique for a Conscious Infant Who is Choking: Towards a More Universal Skill. *Int. J. First Aid Educ.* **2024**, *7*, 1–11. [CrossRef]
36. Miyoshi, T.; Endo, H.; Yamamoto, H.; Shimada, K.; Kumamaru, H.; Ichihara, N.; Miyachi, Y.; Miyata, H. Long-term prognosis and clinical course of choking-induced cardiac arrest in patients without the return of spontaneous circulation at hospital arrival: A population-based community study from the Shizuoka Kokuho Database. *BMC Emerg. Med.* **2022**, *22*, 120, Erratum in: *BMC Emerg. Med.* **2022**, *22*, 157. [CrossRef]
37. Dunne, C.L.; Viguers, K.; Osman, S.; Queiroga, A.C.; Szpilman, D.; Peden, A.E. A 2-year prospective evaluation of airway clearance devices in foreign body airway obstructions. *Resusc. Plus* **2023**, *16*, 100496. [CrossRef]
38. Dunne, C.L.; Peden, A.E.; Queiroga, A.C.; Gomez Gonzalez, C.; Valesco, B.; Szpilman, D. A systematic review on the effectiveness of anti-choking suction devices and identification of research gaps. *Resuscitation* **2020**, *153*, 219–226. [CrossRef]
39. Abbas, A.; Bukhari, S.I.; Ahmad, F. Knowledge of first aid and basic life support amongst medical students: A comparison between trained and un-trained students. *J. Pak. Med. Assoc.* **2011**, *61*, 613–616.
40. Greif, R.; Lockey, A.; Breckwoldt, J.; Carmona, F.; Conaghan, P.; Kuzovlev, A.; Pflanzl-Knizacek, L.; Sari, F.; Shammet, S.; Scapigliati, A.; et al. European Resuscitation Council Guidelines 2021: Education for resuscitation. *Resuscitation* **2021**, *161*, 388–407. [CrossRef]
41. Kasem, A.; Abuhammad, S. Pediatric Basic Life Support among Nursing Students in Jordan: Stimulation-Based Education. *Open J. Nurs.* **2022**, *16*, e2208110. [CrossRef]

healthcare

MDPI

Article

What Mistakes Can Be Made When Performing the Electrical Cardioversion Procedure?—Analysis of Emergency Medical Team Performance during the Championships in Emergency Medicine

Michał Ćwiertnia [1,2,*], Mieczysław Dutka [3], Piotr Białoń [1], Michał Szlagor [1], Arkadiusz Stasicki [1], Monika Mikulska [1], Maciej B. Hajduga [3], Rafał Bobiński [3], Marek Kawecki [1] and Tomasz Ilczak [1,2]

1 Department of Emergency Medicine, Faculty of Health Sciences, University of Bielsko-Biala, Willowa 2, 43-309 Bielsko-Biała, Poland; pbialon@ubb.edu.pl (P.B.); mszlagor@ubb.edu.pl (M.S.); astasicki@ubb.edu.pl (A.S.); mmikulska@ubb.edu.pl (M.M.); mkawecki@ubb.edu.pl (M.K.); tilczak@ubb.edu.pl (T.I.)

2 European Pre-Hospital Research Network, Nottingham NG11 8NS, UK

3 Department of Biochemistry and Molecular Biology, Faculty of Health Sciences, University of Bielsko-Biala, Willowa 2, 43-309 Bielsko-Biała, Poland; mdutka@ubb.edu.pl (M.D.); mbhajduga@ubb.edu.pl (M.B.H.); rbobinski@ubb.edu.pl (R.B.)

* Correspondence: mcwiertnia@ubb.edu.pl

Abstract: Background: Medical personnel carrying out electrical cardioversion (EC) procedures must remember to have the R-wave sync mode switched on, use the correct energy and maintain personal safety. The defibrillators used by medical response teams most often switch out of cardioversion mode once a shock is delivered. Therefore, this mode must be switched on again before subsequent shocks are delivered. The main aim of the study was to assess the ability of emergency medical teams participating in emergency medicine championships to perform EC. Methods: The research was a retrospective observational study and was based on an analysis of the evaluation sheets from two tasks simulating the management of a patient with unstable tachycardia conducted during the International Winter Emergency Medicine Championships. Three-person teams consisting of paramedics and representing the Polish emergency services were included in the study. The team representing the championship organiser and the few foreign teams participating in the competition were excluded from the study. Results: The decision to conduct EC was taken by 36 teams (83.72%) in 2015 and 27 teams (87.10%) in 2019. In both editions of the championships, during consecutive shocks, the percentage of actions performed correctly decreased significantly—switching on synchronisation mode in 2015 (94.4%, 83.33%, 72.22%) and in 2019 (100%, 88.89%, 81.48%); correct energies in 2015 (91.67%, 80.56%, 77.78%) and in 2019 (92.59%, 85.19%, 81.48%); shocks in a safe manner in 2015 (94.44%, 94.44%, 91.67%) and in 2019 (100%, 96.30%, 96.30%). Conclusions: Teams participating in the assessed tasks in a significant majority of cases correctly qualified the patient for EC, and correctly carried out the actions required for this procedure. It is of particular note that with every subsequent shock, the percentage of shocks carried out without the sync mode increased significantly.

Keywords: cardiopulmonary resuscitation; electric cardioversion; advanced life support

1. Introduction

Electrotherapy is one of the most important elements in treating patients in a life-threatening condition. The procedures connected to electrotherapy conducted by members of emergency medical response teams (MRTs) include defibrillation, transcutaneous pacing and EC [1,2]. The EC procedure is the key element in the treatment of patients with unstable tachycardia [3,4]. Correctly conducting this procedure involves ensuring personal safety, using the correct energies and enabling the R-wave sync mode. Maintaining safety is ensured by removing open sources of oxygen to a safe distance, as well as ensuring that nobody touches the patient. The appropriate shock energy depends on the type of heart rhythm and on the number of shocks delivered. EC conducted without sync mode bears the risk of delivering a shock during the relative refractory period of the heart and inducing ventricular fibrillation (VF) [3–7].

The decision to perform EC should always be preceded by a thorough assessment of the patient's condition. This is due to the differences in the management to be undertaken when the patient is or is not showing signs of haemodynamic instability [3,4]. According to European Resuscitation Council (ERC) guidelines, haemodynamic instability can be indicated by symptoms such as shock, syncope, myocardial ischaemia and severe heart failure. In patients with these symptoms, immediate EC is recommended [3].

Even a fully correct EC procedure carries the risk of causing a sudden cardiac arrest in the patient [4,8]. For this reason, the manufacturers of defibrillators usually programme their devices so that the sync mode automatically switches off after EC is carried out [9]. This makes it possible to immediately carry out defibrillation if necessary [7,9]. This situation requires the medical personnel to switch on sync mode again before every subsequent EC attempt [9].

Improving the knowledge and skills of MRTs can be achieved through participation in emergency medicine championships. Thanks to this type of event, the participants can practise treating patients in a variety of life-threatening conditions, and the organisers can demonstrate what the most common mistakes made by team members are [10]. Since 2006, the Bielsko Emergency Services in Poland have organised the International Winter Championships in Emergency Medicine. Three-person medical response teams from Poland take part in the championships, as well as guest teams invited from abroad.

The main aim of the study was to assess the ability of emergency medical teams participating in the International Winter Emergency Medicine Championships to perform EC. The authors assessed the teams' ability to recognise the indications for this procedure, the correctness of its performance and the subsequent management when it was found to be ineffective.

2. Materials and Methods

This research was a retrospective observational study and was conducted on the basis of detailed analysis of assessment cards for tasks carried out during the International Winter Championships in Emergency Medicine in the years 2013–2023. In these years, tasks related to cardiopulmonary resuscitation were prepared and carried out by European Resuscitation Council (ERC) advanced life support instructors. During this period, in 2015 and 2019, there were two tasks involving simulated treatment of a patient with unstable tachycardia. Three-person teams consisting of paramedics and representing the Polish emergency services from all over the country participated in the championships. All of these teams were included in the study. Of the Polish teams, only the organiser's team, which was not included in the championship's generic classification, was excluded from the study. Foreign teams were also excluded from the study, as only a total of three such three-person teams participated in the championships in 2015 and 2019. Teams taking part in the championships were previously registered by the directors of individual units. According to the regulations, only persons currently employed in a given unit could participate. The people preparing and conducting the tasks were in no way connected to any of the championship participants.

The tasks analysed consisted of a ten-minute simulated scenario with an adult with unstable tachycardia. In 2015, the scenario involved a patient with a history of paroxysmal atrial fibrillation, whose symptoms suddenly appeared immediately before the team was called. This patient was unconscious with shock symptoms and features of heart failure. In the 2019 scenario, the same symptoms indicative of hemodynamic instability were present in a patient with ventricular tachycardia.

The procedures were carried out on a MegaCode Kelly mannequin from the firm Laerdal. The assessment cards used by the judges were constructed so as to assess the compliance of the procedures with the then ERC guidelines. Information about the fact that tasks were to be assessed according to ERC guidelines was included in the official championships regulations and participants were also reminded of this before the tasks began. In the analysed tasks, the judges assessed: the decision of the necessity to conduct EC, the enabling of sync mode before every shock, the shock energies, the size of the electrodes/paddles used, personal safety during the shocks, and the administration of amiodarone after the third ineffective shock—the dose, dilution, route and time of administration.

Among the teams who took the decision regarding the necessity of conducting EC, the judges assessed whether the defibrillator was in sync mode before every subsequent shock—in both editions of the championships, all teams used biphasic devices in which this mode was automatically disabled after a shock was delivered. The assessment of the shock energies was based on the then ERC guidelines, as well as on scientific research that the guidelines referred to. In the task, in both 2015 and 2019, the same values were adopted as correct for subsequent shocks. The first shock should have been delivered with an energy of 120–150 J, the second with a higher energy (higher than the first, but not the maximum), and the third on the maximum energy of a given device. Team members should have used paddles/electrodes dedicated for adults. With every shock, it was noted whether any members of the team were touching the patient, and whether open sources of oxygen were removed to a safe distance. After the third ineffective shock, the teams should have begun to administer 300 mg of amiodarone intravenously/intraosseously diluted in 5% glucose within 10–20 min.

For the statistical analysis of the results, the adopted level of significance was $p = 0.05$. In order to test for possible significant differences between the activities covered in the study areas performed at subsequent shocks (enabling sync mode for subsequent shocks, the use of the correct energies for subsequent shocks and the delivery of subsequent shocks in a safe manner), the non-parametric Friedman ANOVA test was used. To precisely determine between which shocks there were significant differences in the individual activities studied, a Bonferroni post hoc test was performed—pairwise comparison. The calculations were made in the R statistical environment version 3.6.0, PSPP version 2.0.0 software and MS Office 2019.

3. Results

The research carried out showed that a total of 74 three-person teams representing Polish emergency services took part in both editions of the championship (43 teams in 2015 and 31 teams in 2019).

Table 1 presents the number and percentage of teams that carried out individual actions correctly in the years 2015 and 2019.

Table 1. Studied actions carried out correctly by MRT members in the years 2015 and 2019.

	2015		2019	
	n	%	*n*	%
Decision of the necessity to conduct EC	36	83.72	27	87.10
Enabling cardioversion mode before 1st shock	34	94.44	27	100
Enabling cardioversion mode before 2nd shock	30	83.33	24	88.89
Enabling cardioversion mode before 3rd shock	26	72.22	22	81.48
1st shock energy	33	91.67	25	92.59
2nd shock energy	29	80.56	23	85.19
3rd shock energy	28	77.78	22	81.48

Table 1. *Cont.*

	2015		2019	
	n	%	*n*	%
Size of paddles/electrodes during 1st shock	36	100	27	100
Size of paddles/electrodes during 2nd shock	36	100	27	100
Size of paddles/electrodes during 3rd shock	36	100	27	100
Personal safety during 1st shock	34	94.44	27	100
Personal safety during 2nd shock	34	94.44	26	96.30
Personal safety during 3rd shock	33	91.67	26	96.30
Decision to administer amiodarone	30	83.33	23	83.87
Amiodarone dose	28	93.33	22	95.65
Amiodarone administering route	30	100	23	100
Time of administering amiodarone	26	86.67	21	91.30
Amiodarone dilution	29	96.67	23	100

n—number of teams.

Table 2 below present difference between the percentage of enabling sync mode for subsequent shocks.

Table 2. Difference between the percentage of enabling sync mode for subsequent shocks.

	χ^2	df	*p*	M	SD	Min	Max	Me
1st shock	98.00	2	<0.001	96.82	2.77	94.44	100.00	94.44
2nd shock				85.74	2.78	83.33	88.89	83.33
3rd shock				76.94	4.67	72.22	81.48	81.48

χ^2—test statistic; df—degrees of freedom; *p*—statistical significance; M—mean; SD—standard deviation; Min—minimum; Max—maximum, Me—median.

The research showed statistically significant differences between the percentage of enabling sync mode for subsequent shocks ($p < 0.05$). It was shown that the correctness of enabling sync mode was decreased significantly with each successive shock. The results are illustrated in Figure 1.

Table 3 below presents the difference between the percentage of use of the correct energies for subsequent shocks.

Table 3. Difference between the percentage of use of the correct energies for subsequent shocks.

	χ^2	df	*p*	M	SD	Min	Max	Me
1st shock	100.00	2	<0.001	92.07	0.46	91.67	92.59	91.67
2nd shock				82.61	2.32	80.56	85.19	80.56
3rd shock				79.41	1.86	77.78	81.48	77.78

χ^2—test statistic; df—degrees of freedom; *p*—statistical significance; M—mean; SD—standard deviation; Min—minimum; Max—maximum; Me—median.

The research showed statistically significant differences between the percentage of use of the correct energies for subsequent shocks ($p < 0.05$). It was shown that the use of the correct energy decreased significantly with each successive shock. The results are illustrated in Figure 2.

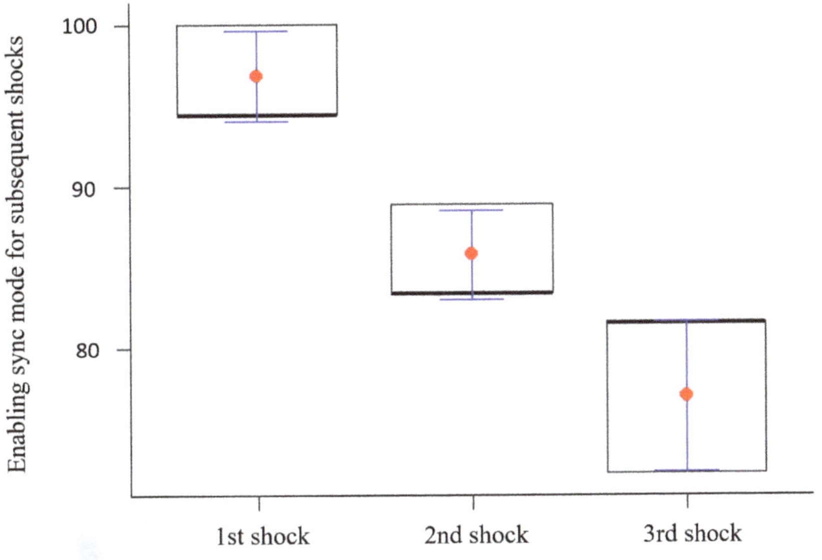

Figure 1. Enabling sync mode for subsequent shocks.

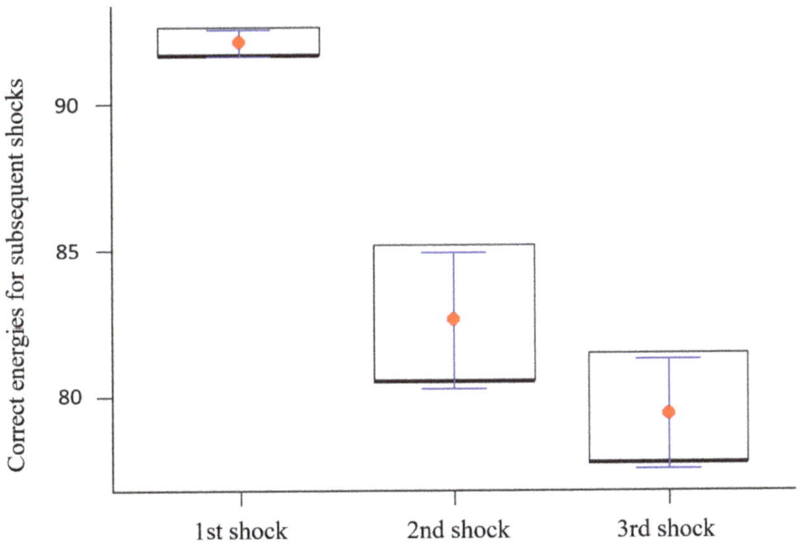

Figure 2. Correct energies for subsequent shocks.

Table 4 below present difference between the percentage of delivering subsequent shocks in a safe manner.

The research showed a statistically significant difference between the percentage of delivering subsequent shocks in a safe manner. ($p < 0.05$). It was shown that delivering subsequent shocks in a safe manner decreased significantly with each successive shock. The results are illustrated in Figure 3.

Table 4. Difference between the percentage of delivering subsequent shocks in a safe manner.

	χ^2	df	p	M	SD	Min	Max	Me
1st shock	88.92	2	<0.001	96.90	2.79	94.44	100.00	94.44
2nd shock				95.25	0.93	94.44	96.30	94.44
3rd shock				93.71	2.32	91.67	96.30	91.67

χ^2—test statistic; df—degrees of freedom; p—statistical significance; M—mean; SD—standard deviation; Min—minimum; Max—maximum; Me—median.

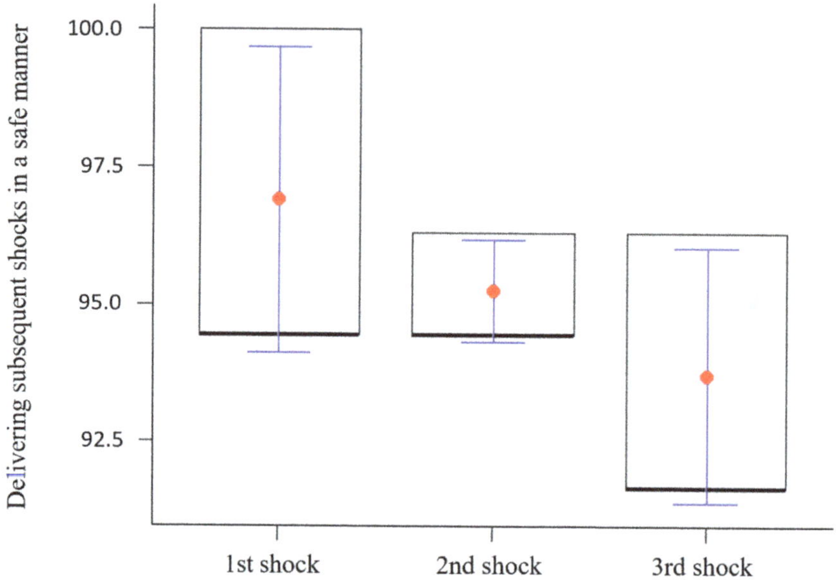

Figure 3. Delivering subsequent shocks in a safe manner.

4. Discussion

In patients with unstable tachycardia, it is necessary to implement the appropriate means of treatment. According to ERC guidelines, this involves immediate use of EC [3]. Our research has shown that, based on the patient's condition, the majority of the teams assessed took the correct decision on the necessity of conducting EC. In 2015, such a decision was taken by 83.72% of the teams, and in 2019 by 87.10%. In one study assessing the skills of 136 paramedics in performing EC, similar results were obtained. The study showed that the correct decision to perform electrical cardioversion was made in 88.7% of cases [11]. Numerous scientific studies have shown [12–15] that this type of management in a patient with unstable tachycardia results in a high probability of a quick return to sinus rhythm.

Correct implementation of EC should be synchronised with the R waves. For this reason, members of MRTs should ensure that the sync mode is enabled before every subsequent shock [3,9,16]. Our research has demonstrated that with subsequent shocks there was a significant increase in the number of situations where synchronisation was not enabled. This situation was most certainly directly influenced by the fact that all teams participating in the championships used devices in which the sync mode was automatically disabled after a shock was delivered. Al Duhailib et al. [9] describe how the automatic disabling of the sync mode makes it possible to immediately conduct defibrillation if the shock induces VF. Our research has shown, however, that this can increase the risk that for subsequent shocks MRT members can forget to switch this mode back on again. Situations in which medical personnel, while treating a patient with tachycardia, forgot to turn on synchronisation mode again after an earlier shock are described in the literature [17]. Such procedural errors can lead to a shock being delivered during the heart's relative refractory period and induce VF [3,18].

According to ERC guidelines, the shock energies for EC should be dependent on the type of heart rhythm and on which subsequent shock is being delivered [1,3]. According to the guidelines [19], in both tasks teams should have delivered the first shock at an energy in the range between 120 and 150 J, and the second shock energy should have been increased so that the third shock was delivered at the maximum energy. Our research has shown that a considerable majority of the teams in both editions of the championships delivered shocks at the correct energies. One survey, conducted in Poland in the form of a questionnaire among paramedics and nurses working in emergency medical teams, showed significantly worse results in terms of knowledge of the EC procedure. These studies showed that only 43.79% of the participants correctly indicated what the shock energy should be during the first EC attempt [20]. In our research, the percentage of correct energies during the first EC attempt was 91.67% in 2015 and 92.59% in 2019. However, it should be noted that during the championship team members had the opportunity to consult with each other before performing individual activities which may have made it easier for them to choose the correct energy. According to some studies [21,22], using the correct shock energies during the EC procedure increases the chances of restoring sinus rhythm.

Shocks delivered during EC should be carried out with the use of paddles or electrodes of an appropriate size [23–25]. Paddles or electrodes intended for paediatric patients should not be used for this purpose for adults [26,27]. This research has shown that the teams always used the correct size of paddles/electrodes in both the analysed tasks. As demonstrated in research papers [26,28], the use of the correct size of paddles or electrodes in this way reduces chest impedance, and therefore increases the chances of delivering an effective shock.

A key element of conducting EC is ensuring the personal safety of the team members [3,4]. Studies have described cases in which patients [29,30] or medical personnel [29,31] have sustained serious injury during electrical shocks. Soar et al. [3] describe how during shocks care must be taken to ensure that no-one is touching the patient and that any oxygen is removed to a safe distance. Our research has shown that teams delivered shocks without due regard for safety in only a minimal percentage of cases. According to the remarks entered by the judges onto assessment cards, these cases mainly amounted to a failure to move an oxygen source to a safe distance. Such behaviour can result in the patient and team members suffering burns [29,31]. A system of regular training can be helpful in eliminating such significant errors. As scientific studies have shown, a short time after training, medical personnel lose knowledge [32,33] and confidence [34] in performing the EC procedure. This situation may also be influenced by the fact that some medical personnel, including EMS personnel, perform this procedure quite infrequently. In their study, Sokolowski et al. [20] showed that as many as 65.09% of the paramedics and nurses working in the EMSs in southwestern Poland had never performed EC. Therefore, systematic participation in training courses on EC [33,34] and especially those in which the use of manual defibrillators is discussed in detail [32] can significantly reduce the number of errors that occur when performing this procedure.

If three attempts at EC on a patient with unstable tachycardia turn out to be ineffective, 300 mg of amiodarone diluted in 5% glucose should be administered intravenously or intraosseously within 10–20 min [3]. Our research has shown that the decision to administer amiodarone was taken by 83.33% of the teams in 2015 and 83.87% of the teams in 2019. These teams always administered the medicine using the correct route and in the vast majority of cases in the correct dose and correct dilution. Another study assessing the knowledge of EMS personnel showed that only 66.86% of them could indicate the correct dose of amiodarone to be given in this situation [20]. In the case of our own study, the correct dose of amiodarone was given by 93.33% of the teams in 2015 and 95.65% in 2019. The implementation by the teams of pharmacological cardioversion in this way is a procedure recommended by the ERC for patients with unstable tachycardia in situations when EC is shown to be ineffective [3].

The results of our study, combined with those of other authors [11,17,20,32–34], may indicate a real existing problem associated with performing the EC procedure. Therefore, special emphasis should be placed on the proper education of paramedics and then systematically training those already working in EMS. As authors, we can propose the introduction into the protocol and recommendations of scientific societies of the principle of confirmation in the form: "Say it loud and say it twice"—where each member of the team checks and confirms the fact that the correct energy is set, synchronisation is turned on and safety is maintained.

The authors of the study are aware of some of its limitations. First of all, the results obtained from this study come from a time when ERC guidelines for the treatment of patients with unstable atrial fibrillation differed from those currently recommended. Another limitation is that the paper does not present descriptive statistics of the study group, as such information was not collected by the championship organisers. The study was conducted in a group of paramedics, so in the future it is necessary to expand it to include a group of doctors and nurses. A limitation of the study is probably also the fact that the participants of the championship were probably chosen as representatives of their EMS units to obtain the best possible result, so they may have had above-average knowledge and skills.

5. Conclusions

Our research based on simulated scenarios has shown that the teams in most cases used the correct management method for selecting energy, enabling the synchronisation mode and maintaining safety when performing the EC procedure. A way to eliminate errors that occur in this area can be systematic training, directed especially to paramedics who rarely perform this procedure. Particularly noteworthy is the fact that with every subsequent shock, there was a significant increase in the percentage of cases of shocks delivered without the use of sync mode. As a result, the study authors suggest that it should be considered that defibrillators be programmed so that the devices remain in sync mode after shocks are delivered. However, this situation requires additional research to assess the effect of sync mode not being disabled on the time when defibrillation can be conducted if EC induces VF.

Author Contributions: M.Ć.—conceptualisation, data curation, formal analysis, investigation, methodology, project administration, resources, supervision, validation, visualisation, writing—original draft, writing—review and editing, supervision; M.D.—formal analysis, methodology, visualisation; P.B.—data curation, formal analysis, validation; M.S.—data curation, formal analysis, investigation; A.S.—data curation, formal analysis, investigation; M.M.—supervision; M.B.H.—supervision; R.B.—supervision; M.K.—supervision, T.I.—data curation, formal analysis, methodology, supervision. All authors have read and agreed to the published version of the manuscript.

Funding: This research received no external funding.

Institutional Review Board Statement: The study was conducted in accordance with the Helsinki Declaration and approved by the Ethics Committee of the University of Bielsko-Biala (Decision No. 2023/4/19/E/22, decision received on 20 April 2023).

Informed Consent Statement: The data collected for analysis do not allow for the identification of participants in any way, nor do they violate their legal and ethical rights.

Data Availability Statement: The datasets used and/or analysed during the current study are available from the corresponding author on reasonable request.

Conflicts of Interest: The authors declare no conflicts of interest.

References

1. Perkins, G.D.; Grasner, J.T.; Semeraro, F.; Olasveengen, T.; Soar, J.; Lott, C.; Van de Voorde, P.; Madar, J.; Zideman, D.; Mentzelopoulos, S.; et al. European Resuscitation Council Guidelines 2021: Executive summary. *Resuscitation* **2021**, *161*, 1–60. [CrossRef] [PubMed]
2. Merchant, R.M.; Topjian, A.A.; Panchal, A.R.; Cheng, A.; Aziz, K.; Berg, K.M.; Lavonas, E.J.; Magid, D.J. Part 1: Executive Summary: 2020 American Heart Association Guidelines for Cardiopulmonary Resuscitation and Emergency Cardiovascular Care. *Circulation* **2020**, *142* (Suppl. S2), 337–357. [CrossRef] [PubMed]
3. Soar, J.; Böttiger, B.W.; Carli, P.; Couper, K.; Deakin, C.D.; Djärv, T.; Lott, C.; Olasveengen, T.; Paal, P.; Pellis, T.; et al. European Resuscitation Council Guidelines 2021: Adult advanced life support. *Resuscitation* **2021**, *161*, 115–151.
4. Panchal, A.R.; Bartos, J.A.; Cabañas, J.G.; Donnino, M.W.; Drennan, I.R.; Hirsch, K.G.; Kudenchuk, P.J.; Kurz, M.C.; Lavonas, E.J.; Morley, P.T.; et al. Part 3: Adult Basic and Advanced Life Support: 2020 American Heart Association Guidelines for Cardiopulmonary Resuscitation and Emergency Cardiovascular Care. *Circulation* **2020**, *142* (Suppl. S2), 366–468. [CrossRef] [PubMed]
5. Brandes, A.; Crijns, H.J.G.M.; Rienstra, M.; Kirchhof, P.; Grove, E.L.; Pedersen, K.B.; Van Gelder, I.C. Cardioversion of atrial fibrillation and atrial flutter revisited: Current evidence and practical guidance for a common procedure. *Europace* **2020**, *22*, 1149–1161. [CrossRef] [PubMed]
6. Nguyen, S.T.; Belley-Côté, E.P.; Ibrahim, O.; Um, K.J.; Lengyel, A.; Adli, T.; Qiu, Y.; Wong, M.; Sibilio, S.; Benz, A.P.; et al. Techniques improving electrical cardioversion success for patients with atrial fibrillation: A systematic review and meta-analysis. *Europace* **2023**, *25*, 318–330. [CrossRef]
7. Goyal, A.; Sciammarella, J.C.; Chhabra, L.; Singhal, M. Synchronized Electrical Cardioversion. 2023 Mar 27. In *StatPearls [Internet]*; StatPearls Publishing: Treasure Island, FL, USA, 2024.
8. Bonfanti, L.; Annovi, A.; Sanchis-Gomar, F.; Saccenti, C.; Meschi, T.; Ticinesi, A.; Cervellin, G. Effectiveness and safety of electrical cardioversion for acute-onset atrial fibrillation in the emergency department: A real-world 10-year single center experience. *Clin. Exp. Emerg. Med.* **2019**, *6*, 64–69. [CrossRef]
9. Al Duhailib, Z.; Trusz-Gluza, M.; Jankowski, M. Electrical Cardioversion. McMaster Textbook of Internal Medicine. Kraków: Medycyna Praktyczna. Available online: https://empendium.com/mcmtextbook/chapter/B31.IV.24.63 (accessed on 21 August 2024).
10. Smart, J.R.; Kranz, K.; Carmona, F.; Lindner, T.W.; Newton, A. Does real-time objective feedback and competition improve performance and quality in manikin CPR training-a prospective observational study from several European EMS. *Scand. J. Trauma Resusc. Emerg. Med.* **2015**, *23*, 79. [CrossRef]
11. Hakyemez, F.; Kara, H. Assesment of the Knowledge and Skills of Paramedics Working in Prehospital Health Services on Making a Decision for and Applying Defibrillation and Cardioversion. *Anatol. J. Emerg. Med.* **2021**, *4*, 43–48.
12. Stiell, I.G.; Eagles, D.; Nemnom, M.J.; Brown, E.; Taljaard, M.; RAFF Investigators; Archambault, P.M.; Birnie, D.; Borgundvaag, B.; Clark, G.; et al. Adverse Events Associated with Electrical Cardioversion in Patients with Acute Atrial Fibrillation and Atrial Flutter. *Can. J. Cardiol.* **2021**, *37*, 1775–1782.
13. Fried, A.M.; Strout, T.D.; Perron, A.D. Electrical cardioversion for atrial fibrillation in the emergency department: A large single-center experience. *Am. J. Emerg. Med.* **2021**, *42*, 115–120. [CrossRef]
14. Strzelczyk, T.A.; Kaplan, R.M.; Medler, M.; Knight, B.P. Outcomes associated with electrical cardioversion for atrial fibrillation when performed autonomously by an advanced practice provider. *JACC Clin. Electrophysiol.* **2017**, *3*, 1447–1452. [CrossRef]
15. Prasai, P.; Shrestha, D.B.; Saad, E.; Trongtorsak, A.; Adhikari, A.; Gaire, S.; Oli, P.R.; Shtembari, J.; Adhikari, P.; Sedhai, Y.R.; et al. Electric Cardioversion vs. Pharmacological with or without Electric Cardioversion for Stable New-Onset Atrial Fibrillation: A Systematic Review and Meta-Analysis. *J. Clin. Med.* **2023**, *12*, 1165. [CrossRef] [PubMed]
16. Schmidt, A.S.; Lauridsen, K.G.; Adelborg, K.; Torp, P.; Bach, L.F.; Jepsen, S.M.; Hornung, N.; Deakin, C.D.; Rickers, H.; Løfgren, B. Cardioversion Efficacy Using Pulsed Biphasic or Biphasic Truncated Exponential Waveforms: A Randomized Clinical Trial. *J. Am. Heart Assoc.* **2017**, *6*, e004853. [CrossRef] [PubMed]
17. Pchejetski, D.; Alam, T.; Alshaker, H. Unsynchronised Cardioversion as a Cause of Ventricular Tachycardia in a Patient with Atrial Fibrillation. *Cardiol. Case Rep.* **2020**, *1*, 2. [CrossRef]
18. Ikeda, S.; An, Y.; Yanagisawa, M.; Ishigami, K.; Aono, Y.; Doi, K.; Ishii, M.; Iguchi, M.; Ogawa, H.; Masunaga, N.; et al. Iatrogenic ventricular fibrillation caused by inappropriately synchronized cardioversion in a patient with pre-excited atrial fibrillation: A case report. *J. Cardiol. Cases* **2020**, *23*, 31–34. [CrossRef] [PubMed]
19. Soar, J.; Nolan, J.P.; Böttiger, B.W.; Perkins, G.D.; Lott, C.; Carli, P.; Pellis, T.; Sandroni, C.; Skrifvars, M.B.; Smith, G.B.; et al. European Resuscitation Council Guidelines for Resuscitation 2015: Section 3. Adult advanced life support. *Resuscitation* **2015**, *95*, 100–147. [CrossRef] [PubMed]
20. Sokolowski, M.; Wawrzynska, M. Knowledge of and attitudes to emergency tachyarrhythmia treatment among paramedics and nurses. *Disaster Emerg. Med. J.* **2019**, *4*, 9–13. [CrossRef]
21. Patti, L.; Ashurst, J.V. Supraventricular Tachycardia. [Updated 2023 Aug 7]. In *StatPearls [Internet]*; StatPearls Publishing: Treasure Island, FL, USA, 2024. Available online: https://www.ncbi.nlm.nih.gov/books/NBK441972/ (accessed on 1 August 2024).
22. Darrat, Y.; Leung, S.; Elayi, L.; Parrott, K.; Ogunbayo, G.; Kotter, J.; Sorrell, V.; Gupta, V.; Anaya, P.; Morales, G.; et al. A stepwise external cardioversion protocol for atrial fibrillation to maximize acute success rate. *Europace* **2023**, *25*, 828–834. [CrossRef]

23. Pal-Jakab, A.; Nagy, B.; Kiss, B.; Zima, E. The Influence of Transthoracic Impedance on Electrical Cardioversion and Defibrillation: Current Data [Internet]. In *Updates on Cardiac Defibrillation, Cardioversion and AED Development*; IntechOpen: London, UK, 2024. [CrossRef]
24. Vostrikov, V.A.; Razumov, K.V.; Gorbunov, B.B. Impact of Electrode Size on the Efficacy of Electrical Cardioversion for Paroxysmal Atrial Fibrillation. *Biomed. Eng.* **2016**, *50*, 179–183. [CrossRef]
25. Roh, S.Y.; Ahn, J.; Lee, K.N.; Baek, Y.S.; Kim, D.H.; Lee, D.I.; Shim, J.; Choi, J.I.; Kim, Y.H. The Impact of Personal Thoracic Impedance on Electrical Cardioversion in Patients with Atrial Arrhythmias. *Medicina* **2021**, *57*, 618. [CrossRef] [PubMed]
26. Van de Voorde, P.; Turner, N.M.; Djakow, J.; de Lucas, N.; Martinez-Mejias, A.; Biarent, D.; Bingham, R.; Brissaud, O.; Hoffmann, F.; Johannesdottir, G.B.; et al. European Resuscitation Council Guidelines 2021: Paediatric Life Support. *Resuscitation* **2021**, *161*, 327–387. [CrossRef] [PubMed]
27. Heyer, Y.; Baumgartner, D.; Baumgartner, C.A. Systematic Review of the Transthoracic Impedance during Cardiac Defibrillation. *Sensors* **2022**, *22*, 2808. [CrossRef]
28. Yin, R.T.; Taylor, T.G.; de Graaf, C.; Ekkel, M.M.; Chapman, F.W.; Koster, R.W. Automated external defibrillator electrode size and termination of ventricular fibrillation in out-of-hospital cardiac arrest. *Resuscitation* **2023**, *185*, 109754. [CrossRef] [PubMed]
29. Beebeejaun, A.; Howard, R. Dangers of defibrillation in flight. *J. Australas. Soc. Aerosp. Med.* **2020**, *11*, 1–4. [CrossRef]
30. Koda, E.K. Lumbar Compression Fracture Caused by Cardioversion. *Am. J. Case Rep.* **2020**, *21*, e927064. [CrossRef]
31. Gibbs, W.; Eisenberg, M.; Damon, S.K. Dangers of defibrillation: Injuries to emergency personnel during patient resuscitation. *Am. J. Emerg. Med.* **1990**, *8*, 101–104. [CrossRef]
32. Siebert, J.N.; Glangetas, A.; Grange, M.; Haddad, K.; Courvoisier, D.S.; Lacroix, L. Impact of blended learning on manual defibrillator's use: A simulation-based randomized trial. *Nurs. Crit. Care* **2022**, *27*, 501–511. [CrossRef]
33. Kowalski, C.; Boulesteix, A.L.; Harendza, S. Effective methods to enhance medical students' cardioversion and transcutaneous cardiac pacing skills retention—A prospective controlled study. *BMC Med. Educ.* **2022**, *22*, 417. [CrossRef]
34. Smith, A.W.; Elliott, J.O.; Gable, B.D. Simulation Improves Internal Medicine Resident Confidence With Defibrillation, Cardioversion, and Transcutaneous Pacemaker Use. *Cureus* **2021**, *13*, e16648. [CrossRef]

2.7. Statistical Analysis

The adopted level of significance was $p = 0.05$, according to which results with $p < 0.05$ represent significant dependencies between the variables. Variables expressed on an ordinal or nominal level were analysed using tests based on the chi-squared distribution. In the case of 2×2 tables, continuity correction was used, whereas if the conditions of using the chi-squared test were not fulfilled, the precise Fisher test was applied with extension for tables larger than 2×2. Parametric tests (ANOVA variance analysis) or their non-parametric equivalents (the Kruskal–Wallis test) were used to analyse the quantitative variables divided into groups. The selection of the tests was conducted on the basis of the distribution of the variables, which was verified using the Shapiro–Wilk test. Verification of relationships between the variables was conducted using polynomial logistic regression analysis. Calculations were carried out in the R statistical environment version 3.6.0, PSPP software (https://www.gnu.org/software/pspp/) and MS Office 2019.

3. Results

The data in Table 1 present the description of the study group by gender and stage of the disease.

The data in Table 2 present a comparison between the clinical assessment and CT image of the severity of a patient's condition. Patients in a mild clinical condition most often had a mild degree of lung damage on the CT image (45.7%), similarly to patients in an average clinical condition (45.2%). Patients in a severe clinical condition most often had an average degree of damage on the CT image. No statistically significant differences were shown ($p > 0.05$), which indicates that at the initial stage of examining a patient, the clinical assessment is comparative to the assessment obtained using CT imaging.

Table 2. Differences in clinical assessments of disease severity with reference to first computed tomography result.

			Clinical Assessment of Stage of Disease			**Test Result**
			Mild Condition	**Average Condition**	**Severe Condition**	
Computed tomography result	Mild condition	N	16	14	3	$\chi^2 = 6.352$ $df = 4$ $p = 0.174$
		%	45.7%	45.2%	15.8%	
	Average condition	N	14	10	10	
		%	40.0%	32.3%	52.6%	
	Severe condition	N	5	7	6	
		%	14.3%	22.6%	31.6%	
Total		N	35	31	19	
		%	100.0%	100.0%	100.0%	

χ^2—test statistic; df—degrees of freedom; N—number; and p—statistical significance.

Table 3 presents the results obtained from laboratory tests in relation to the CT image of lung damage. The data show that upon admittance, BNP, BE and HCO_3^- values, selected due to the degree of lung damage in the CT, differ from one another statistically significantly ($p < 0.05$). For the remainder, the observed differences were not statistically significant. The research demonstrated that along with an increase in the severity of damage to the lungs, there was a statistically insignificant increase in the values of IL6 and LDH, TNF, TGFb1, D-dimer and LAC. People with mild lung damage had minimally higher values of fibrinogen, pH and SpO_2. People with average damage had minimally higher CRP and pCO_2, while people with severe damage had higher PCT.

Table 3. Laboratory test results obtained upon patient admittance to hospital in comparison to assessment of disease severity in the first computed tomography imaging.

Parameter	CT Result	χ^2	*df*	*p*	*Min*	*Max*	*Me*
BNP [pg/mL]	Mild condition	37.18	2	<0.001	0.71	15.05	3.28
	Average condition				6.29	20.47	10.73
	Severe condition				1.38	24.39	15.66
IL6 [pg/mL]	Mild condition	12.06	2	0.055	0.03	41.60	4.07
	Average condition				0.21	534.40	10.58
	Severe condition				2.68	471.60	17.02
LDH [U/L]	Mild condition	17.27	2	0.055	5.90	26.99	11.88
	Average condition				7.74	119.80	13.59
	Severe condition				10.35	38.91	19.80
TNF [pg/mL]	Mild condition	3.19	2	0.202	27.51	6691.00	45.40
	Average condition				33.41	5219.00	49.11
	Severe condition				20.73	769.00	57.44
TGFb1 [pg/mL]	Mild condition	5.30	2	0.071	35.67	430.80	47.08
	Average condition				39.97	681.10	53.26
	Severe condition				44.06	651.90	55.01
D-dimer [ng/mL]	Mild condition	4.58	2	0.101	264.90	31,382.59	874.58
	Average condition				346.89	36,218.18	969.80
	Severe condition				522.50	14,556.26	1830.43
CRP [mg/L]	Mild condition	2.88	2	0.237	15.70	278.00	81.40
	Average condition				4.90	327.00	103.00
	Severe condition				4.90	290.00	89.60
PCT [ng/mL]	Mild condition	0.39	2	0.823	0.02	1.78	0.13
	Average condition				0.02	1.31	0.12
	Severe condition				0.04	0.64	0.15
Trop T [ng/mL]	Mild condition	1.50	2	0.473	0.00	0.05	0.01
	Average condition				0.00	0.09	0.01
	Severe condition				0.00	0.53	0.01
LAC [mg/dL]	Mild condition	0.97	2	0.617	0.76	3.45	1.47
	Average condition				0.85	4.02	1.56
	Severe condition				0.98	3.27	1.69
Fibrinogen [g/L]	Mild condition	0.91	2	0.635	1.09	8.91	7.02
	Average condition				2.35	8.91	6.11
	Severe condition				3.40	8.91	6.79
pH	Mild condition	2.44	2	0.295	7.31	7.56	7.47
	Average condition				7.31	7.56	7.45
	Severe condition				7.36	7.54	7.46
SpO_2 [%]	Mild condition	2.32	2	0.313	53.50	98.50	91.40
	Average condition				46.80	98.90	87.00
	Severe condition				39.50	99.40	90.65
pO_2 [mmHg]	Mild condition	1.73	2	0.421	42.70	138.10	74.30
	Average condition				25.20	155.40	72.50
	Severe condition				19.00	113.20	78.05

Table 3. *Cont.*

Parameter	CT Result	χ^2	*df*	*p*	*Min*	*Max*	*Me*
BE [mmol/L]	Mild condition	6.30	2	0.043	−5.50	8.00	1.75
	Average condition				−5.30	6.60	1.20
	Severe condition				−2.10	8.00	1.85
pCO_2 [mmHg]	Mild condition	0.27	2	83	0.766	37.78	6.24
	Average condition					38.83	7.52
	Severe condition					39.13	5.38
HCO_3 [mmol/L]	Mild condition	5.26	2	83	0.007	24.62	3.95
	Average condition					22.93	4.07
	Severe condition					26.43	3.24

χ^2—test statistic; *df*—degrees of freedom; *p*—statistical significance; *Min*—minimum result; *Max*—maximum result; and *Me*—median.

In order to precisely determine between which groups the differences are statistically significant, a post hoc Bonferroni test was conducted, as well as Tukey's post hoc test —pairwise comparisons. The results of the obtained comparisons are presented in Table 4.

Table 4. Pairwise comparison of statistically significant laboratory diagnostic results in relation to lung damage on computed tomography imaging.

	Computed Tomography Result		*p*	
BNP [pg/mL] [1]	mild	average	<0.001	***
	mild	severe	<0.001	***
	average	severe	0.014	*
BE [mmol/L] [1]	mild	average	0.129	
	mild	severe	1.000	
	average	severe	0.049	*
HCO_3 [mmol/L] [2]	mild	average	0.118	
	mild	severe	0.319	
	average	severe	0.006	**

[1] Bonferroni post hoc test; [2] Tukey's post hoc test; * $p < 0.05$; ** $p < 0.01$; *** $p < 0.001$; and *p*—statistical significance.

Tabel 4 presents pairwise comparisons of laboratory diagnostic parameters obtained upon admittance of the patient to hospital. Statistically significant differences were obtained in every range for type B natriuretic peptide (BNP). It can be seen that the value of this parameter in the case of average lung damage visible on the CT image was statistically significantly greater than in the case of mild damage ($p < 0.05$). Similarly, in the case of severe lung damage, the BNP values were statistically significantly higher than in the case of average damage ($p < 0.05$). Analogically, in the case of comparison between mild damage and severe damage, the BNP values were higher in the case of severe lung damage. In terms of the level of type B natriuretic peptide, it can be seen that an increase in lung damage, and thus more severe COVID-19, is accompanied by a statistically significant rise in BNP values. A BE alkaline deficiency in comparison to the severity of the disease described in the CT increased between the average and severe condition ($p < 0.05$). It can therefore be seen that in the case of severe COVID-19, BE increases statistically significantly in relation to an average condition. Similarly, in the case of the HCO_3^- parameter, statistically significant differences were noted between people with average lung damage and people with severe damage. People with severe lung damage had a statistically significant ($p < 0.05$) higher HCO_3 value than people with average damage.

4. Discussion

Diagnostic difficulties related to identifying the presence of COVID-19 have existed since the beginning of the pandemic. Research is underway to facilitate the issuing of a correct diagnosis, as well as to determine a patient's prognosis and correctly assess their condition in a short time. Such an approach is vital from the point of view of early assessment of a patient's condition upon admittance to hospital, as well as quick identification of the degree of advancement of the disease [10–13]. In many cases, researchers are seeking solutions to this problem by creating new research models based on the assessment of highly varied factors. The basic elements described in the literature are laboratory diagnostics and imaging, demographic factors and the presence of co-existing illnesses [14–16]. Unfortunately, in the current reality, physical examination of patients, on the basis of which clinical conclusions can be drawn about the course of the disease, are replaced with ICT solutions or distance testing and assessment that are often used to give a final diagnosis or to qualify a patient for the appropriate treatment. In their work, Maćkowiak and Gelfman [17,18] clearly draw attention to the fact that technological development and the epidemiological situation should not lead to such a situation in which physical examinations are treated as of secondary importance. Unfortunately, during their literature review, the authors noted difficulties in finding scientific publications indicating the usefulness of a physical examination in assessing and categorising COVID-19 patients. In our research, we made a pioneering attempt to assign patients to the appropriate disease severity group on the basis of a physical examination and the necessary oxygen therapy or ventilation, without the need to conduct imaging diagnostics. The subject of oxygen therapy and ventilation for COVID-19 patients has been broadly described in the literature. In his work, Nair [19] compared the effectiveness of oxygen therapy via NIV and HFNO in relation to the prognosis for patients with severe COVID-19, concluding that he did not obtain an obvious answer as to the advantage of either method. In their work, Menzella et al. [20] proved that the use of non-invasive ventilation decreased the necessity to move patients to the intensive care ward, while Antonelli et al. [21] confirmed that non-invasive ventilation is effective in COVID-19 patients. None of the authors mentioned above made an attempt in their research to use the applied oxygen therapy as an indicator of the severity of COVID-19. In our research, we have shown that examining the patient and qualifying them for the appropriate oxygen therapy can be used as a parameter to indicate the severity of the disease, and as an estimation of the amount of lung area affected by the illness.

In the next stage, the result of the physical examination and the ventilation method used were matched to the laboratory diagnostics parameters. The result obtained clearly indicates differences in the levels of BNP, BE and HCO_3^- depending on the severity of the disease and the amount of lung parenchyma affected by the disease on the CT image. Similar research was presented by Ghelfi AM [22], in which an increase was demonstrated in NT pro-BNP values proportionally to the severity of the condition of the COVID-19 patient. In the same study, the level of troponin T was assessed, which similarly to our study showed no statistically significant differences. Salvatore C et al. [23] compared laboratory results with the severity of lung damage on the CT image. This study was conducted on patients divided into three groups depending on the severity of the disease. On the basis of their results, they showed that CRP, leukocytes, neutrophils, LDH, D-Dimer and troponin values were statistically significantly higher in patients with a more severe condition. In their research, Zhang et al. [24] demonstrated that the level of some inflammatory markers increased along with the severity of the disease. They proved that the level of CRP and PCT increased in severely ill patients, which in our research was not confirmed statistically. Analysing our results in terms of laboratory norms, it can be seen that some parameters increased depending on the severity of the disease and the amount of lung parenchyma affected by the disease, but that these values were not statistically significant for the research model. Considering the results from the perspective of arterial blood gas analysis, it was possible to identify two key elements that indicate the severity of the disease and the degree of lung infection. In the analysed material, a statistically significant increase was observed in BE and HCO_3^-. In their research, Turcato et al. [25] proved there was a rise in pCO_2 and a drop in pO_2 in patients admitted to hospital with severe COVID-19. They correlated these results with CT images and demonstrated statistically significant dependencies. However, our research did not reveal a correlation between changes in pO_2 and pCO2 depending on the severity of the disease. Sanghani et al. [26] showed the presence of respiratory alkalosis and metabolic alkalosis secondary to it. Our research partly confirmed these results and indicated an increase in BE and HCO_3^- parameters, but no significant changes were observed in terms of pH. A careful review of the literature shows that the laboratory markers used in our research model are often used for COVID-19 diagnostics. Physical examination and oxygen therapy are not commonly used to determine the predictive model or to assess the severity of the disease. It must be underlined that previously, nobody had taken the effort to combine these factors and use them as a diagnostic tool. The model developed in this research can be an effective tool for assisting in determining the severity of COVID-19 and the degree to which the lung parenchyma is affected by the disease.

5. Limitations

The main limitation of the research is that it was conducted in only one centre, while to obtained more transparent results, it would be necessary to repeat the research in multiple centres. A limitation is the lack of opportunity to implement the research project in test conditions, caused by the research being conducted in difficult epidemiological conditions. The research model also requires further work so as to avoid loss of data and an amount of research material while the research is in progress.

6. Conclusions

1. On the basis of a physical examination and the applied oxygen therapy, a patient can be assigned to the appropriate group of severity of COVID-19.
2. On the basis of BNP, HCO_3 and BE parameters obtained from arterial blood, a patient can be assigned to the appropriate group of severity of COVID-19.

Author Contributions: Conceptualization, T.I., S.S. and S.B.; methodology, T.I. and S.B.; validation, R.B. and W.W.; formal analysis, M.Ć. and W.W.; investigation, E.O., M.K. (Mirosław Kucharski), T.S., M.J. (Marta Jagosz), A.J., M.W. and M.J. (Marek Jędrzejek); resources, T.I. and S.B.; data curation, W.W., R.B. and M.K. (Mirosław Kucharski); writing—original draft preparation, T.I.; writing—review and editing, T.I, M.D., R.P. and P.K.; supervision, M.K. (Marek Kawecki) and S.B.; project administration, T.I. All authors have read and agreed to the published version of the manuscript.

Funding: This research received no external funding.

Institutional Review Board Statement: Permission for the research was granted by the ethics committee of the Silesian Medical University (No PCN/CBN/0022/KB1/125/I/21/22, 8 February 2022).

Informed Consent Statement: Not applicable.

Data Availability Statement: The data presented in this study are available on request from the corresponding author.

Conflicts of Interest: The authors declare no conflicts of interest.

References

1. Wu, Z.; McGoogan, J.M. Characteristics of and important lessons from the coronavirus disease 2019 (COVID-19) outbreak in China: Summary of a report of 72314 cases from the Chinese center for disease control and prevention. *J. Am. Med. Assoc.* 2020, *in press*. [CrossRef]
2. Ye, Q.; Wang, B.; Mao, J. The pathogenesis and treatment of the 'Cytokine Storm' in COVID-19. *J. Infect.* **2020**, *80*, 607–613. [CrossRef]
3. Inciardi, R.M.; Lupi, L.; Zaccone, G.; Italia, L.; Rafo, M.; Tomasoni, D.; Cani, D.S.; Cerini, M.; Farina, D.; Gavazzi, E.; et al. Cardiac involvement in a patient with coronavirus disease 2019 (COVID-19). *JAMA Cardiol.* **2020**, *5*, 819–824. [CrossRef] [PubMed]
4. Rothan, H.A.; Byrareddy, S.N. The epidemiology and pathogenesis of coronavirus disease (COVID-19) outbreak. *J. Autoimmun.* **2020**, *109*, 102433. [CrossRef]
5. Auener, S.; Kroon, D.; Wackers, E.; Dulmen, S.V.; Jeurissen, P. COVID-19: A Window of Opportunity for Positive Healthcare Reforms. *Int. J. Health Policy Manag.* **2020**, *9*, 419–422. [CrossRef]

6. Shi, H.; Han, X.; Jiang, N.; Cao, Y.; Alwalid, O.; Gu, J.; Fan, Y.; Zheng, C. Radiological findings from 81 patients with COVID-19 pneumonia in Wuhan, China: A descriptive study. *Lancet Infect Dis.* **2020**, *20*, 425–434. [CrossRef] [PubMed]
7. Chung, M.; Bernheim, A.; Mei, X.; Zhang, N.; Huang, M.; Zeng, X.; Cui, J.; Xu, W.; Yang, Y.; Fayad, Z.A.; et al. CT imaging features of 2019 novel coronavirus (2019-nCoV). *Radiology* **2020**, *295*, 202–207. [CrossRef]
8. Jafari, S.; Tabary, M.; Eshraghi, S.; Araghi, F.; Aryannejad, A.; Mohammadnejad, E.; Rasoolinejad, M.; Hajiabdolbaghi, M.; Koochak, H.E.; Ahmadinejad, Z.; et al. CT-scan fndings of COVID-19 pneumonia based on the time elapsed from the beginning of symptoms to the CT imaging evaluation: A descriptive study in Iran. *Rom. J. Intern. Med.* **2020**, *58*, 242–250. [PubMed]
9. Yazdi, N.A.; Ghadery, A.H.; SeyedAlinaghi, S.; Jafari, F.; Jafari, S.; Hasannezad, M.; Koochak, H.E.; Salehi, M.; Manshadi, S.A.D.; Meidani, M.; et al. Predictors of the chest CT score in COVID-19 patients: A cross-sectional study. *Virol. J.* **2021**, *18*, 225. Erratum in *Virol. J.* **2021**, *18*, 241. [CrossRef] [PubMed] [PubMed Central]
10. Wang, D.; Hu, B.; Hu, C.; Zhu, F.; Liu, X.; Zhang, J.; Wang, B.; Xiang, H.; Cheng, Z.; Xiong, Y.; et al. Clinical characteristics of 138 hospitalized patients with 2019 novel coronavirus–infected pneumonia in Wuhan, China. *JAMA* **2020**, *323*, 1061–1069. [CrossRef]
11. Wang, A.Z.; Ehrman, R.; Bucca, A.; Croft, A.; Glober, N.; Holt, D.; Lardaro, T.; Musey, P.; Peterson, K.; Schaffer, J.; et al. Can we predict which COVID-19 patients will need transfer to intensive care within 24 hours of floor admission? *Acad. Emerg. Med.* **2021**, *28*, 511–518. [CrossRef] [PubMed]
12. Berenguer, J.; Borobia, A.M.; Ryan, P.; Rodríguez-Baño, J.; Bellón, J.M.; Jarrín, I.; Carratalà, J.; Pachón, J.; Carcas, A.J.; Yllescas, M.; et al. Development and validation of a prediction model for 30-day mortality in hospitalised patients with COVID-19: The COVID-19 SEIMC score. *Thorax* **2021**, *76*, 920–929. [CrossRef] [PubMed]
13. Ilczak, T.; Micor, A.; Waksmańska, W.; Bobiński, R.; Kawecki, M. Factors which impact the length of hospitalisation and death rate of COVID-19 patients based on initial triage using capillary blood gas tests: A single centre study. *Sci. Rep.* **2022**, *12*, 17458. [CrossRef] [PubMed]
14. Zheng, Y.; Wang, L.; Ben, S. Meta-analysis of chest CT features of patients with COVID-19 pneumonia. *J. Med. Virol.* **2021**, *93*, 241–249. [CrossRef] [PubMed]
15. Safiabadi Tali, S.H.; LeBlanc, J.J.; Sadiq, Z.; Oyewunmi, O.D.; Camargo, C.; Nikpour, B.; Armanfard, N.; Sagan, S.M.; Jahanshahi-Anbuhi, S. Tools and Techniques for Severe Acute Respiratory Syndrome Coronavirus 2 (SARS-CoV-2)/COVID-19 Detection. *Clin. Microbiol. Rev.* **2021**, *34*, e00228-20. [CrossRef]
16. Hippisley-Cox, J.; Coupland, C.A.; Mehta, N.; Keogh, R.H.; Diaz-Ordaz, K.; Khunti, K.; Lyons, R.A.; Kee, F.; Sheikh, A.; Rahman, S.; et al. Risk prediction of COVID-19 related death and hospital admission in adults after COVID-19 vaccination: National prospective cohort study. *BMJ* **2021**, *374*, n2244. Erratum in *BMJ* **2021**, *374*, n2300. [CrossRef] [PubMed] [PubMed Central]
17. Mackowiak, P.A. COVID-19, Telemedicine, and the Demise of the Physician's Touch. *South. Med. J.* **2021**, *114*, 237–238. [CrossRef] [PubMed] [PubMed Central]
18. Gelfman, D.M. Will the Traditional Physical Examination Be Another Casualty of COVID-19? *Am. J. Med.* **2021**, *134*, 299–300. [CrossRef] [PubMed]
19. Nair, P.R.; Haritha, D.; Behera, S.; Kayina, C.A.; Maitra, S.; Anand, R.K.; Ray, B.R.; Soneja, M.; Subramaniam, R.; Baidya, D.K. Comparison of High-Flow Nasal Cannula and Noninvasive Ventilation in Acute Hypoxemic Respiratory Failure Due to Severe COVID-19 Pneumonia. *Respir. Care.* **2021**, *66*, 1824–1830. [CrossRef] [PubMed] [PubMed Central]
20. Menzella, F.; Barbieri, C.; Fontana, M.; Scelfo, C.; Castagnetti, C.; Ghidoni, G.; Ruggiero, P.; Livrieri, F.; Piro, R.; Ghidorsi, L.; et al. Effectiveness of noninvasive ventilation in COVID-19 related-acute respiratory distress syndrome. *Clin. Respir. J.* **2021**, *15*, 779–787. [CrossRef]
21. Antonelli, M.; Conti, G.; Esquinas, A.; Montini, L.; Maggiore, S.M.; Bello, G.; Rocco, M.; Maviglia, R.; Pennisi, M.A.; Gonzalez-Diaz, G.; et al. A multiple-center survey on the use in clinical practice of noninvasive ventilation as a first-line intervention for acute respiratory distress syndrome. *Crit. Care Med.* **2007**, *35*, 18–25. [CrossRef] [PubMed]
22. Ghelfi, A.M.; Sánchez, B.A.; Berbotto, L.A.; Dipaolo, F.R.; Bosque, V.; Velez, L.L.; Cordone, M.A.; Pallero, R.N.; Yiguerimian, L.M.; Kilstein, J.G. Niveles plasmáticos de troponina T y de la fracción aminoterminal del propéptido natriurético cerebral y su relación con mortalidad en COVID-19 [Troponin-T and n-terminal pro-brain type natriuretic peptide plasma levels and its relationship with mortality in COVID-19]. *Hipertens Riesgo Vasc.* **2022**, *39*, 105–113. (In Spanish) [CrossRef] [PubMed] [PubMed Central]
23. Salvatore, C.; Roberta, F.; Angela, L.; Cesare, P.; Alfredo, C.; Giuliano, G.; Giulio, L.; Giuliana, G.; Maria, R.G.; Paola, B.M.; et al. Clinical and laboratory data, radiological structured report findings and quantitative evaluation of lung involvement on baseline chest CT in COVID-19 patients to predict prognosis. *Radiol. Med.* **2021**, *126*, 29–39. Erratum in *Radiol Med.* **2021**. [CrossRef] [PubMed] [PubMed Central]
24. Zhang, J.; Meng, G.; Li, W.; Shi, B.; Dong, H.; Su, Z.; Huang, Q.; Gao, P. Relationship of chest CT score with clinical characteristics of 108 patients hospitalized with COVID-19 in Wuhan, China. *Respir. Res.* **2020**, *21*, 180. [CrossRef] [PubMed] [PubMed Central]
25. Turcato, G.; Panebianco, L.; Zaboli, A.; Scheurer, C.; Ausserhofer, D.; Wieser, A.; Pfeifer, N. Correlation between arterial blood gas and CT volumetry in patients with SARS-CoV-2 in the emergency department. *Int. J. Infect. Dis.* **2020**, *97*, 233–235. [CrossRef]
26. Sanghani, H.; Bansal, S.; Parmar, V.; Shah, R. Study of Arterial Blood Gas Analysis in Moderate-to-Severe COVID-19 Patients. *Cureus* **2022**, *14*, e26715. [CrossRef] [PubMed] [PubMed Central]

healthcare

MDPI

Review

Adult Triage in the Emergency Department: Introducing a Multi-Layer Triage System

Dimitrios Tsiftsis [1,*], Andreas Tasioulis [1] and Dimitrios Bampalis [2]

1 Emergency Department, Nikaia General Hospital, 184 54 Nikaia, Greece; adreastasioulis@gmail.com
2 Emergency Department, General Hospital of Larisa, 413 34 Larisa, Greece; dbabales@yahoo.com
* Correspondence: deltatangogr@yahoo.com

Abstract: Emergency department (ED) triage is the cornerstone of ED operations. Many different triage systems have been proposed and implemented globally. To date, an ideal triage system has not yet been identified. As the burden on EDs rises, with overcrowding being recognized as a universal problem, ED triage needs to be restructured to address this reality. Extensive and critical literature research over the years has identified the strengths and weaknesses of current ED triage implementations. A novel multi-layer triage system was introduced and implemented in Greek Eds, combining the strengths of various triage and early warning systems and scores to minimize under-triage and the adverse downstream effects it creates on patient outcomes. Acknowledging that no triage system can be universally adapted in different settings, the structural concepts of this triage system address most of the triage problems currently reported in the literature.

Keywords: triage; early warning scores; ESI; NEWS; HEART; emergency department

1. Introduction

Emergency department (ED) overcrowding is a global phenomenon that delays diagnostic and therapeutic interventions [1]. This delay might crucially affect patient outcomes [2]. As ED patient volumes increase and even more people endure constantly prolonged waiting times, an accurate triage system becomes vital.

Hospital triage is a process through which healthcare professionals actively try to identify high-acuity patients and prioritize them accordingly. These patients range from critically ill, in need of immediate life-saving interventions, to patients with minor medical problems who are low urgency. The majority of the ED population lies between these two extremes. Both over-triage and under-triage hurt ED flow and patient waiting times. Under-triage might leave a critical patient in the waiting room for a prolonged period leading to severe deterioration. Over-triage will overflow the treatment area with lower acuity patients consuming all available treatment places and resources and thus preventing higher acuity patients from entering in a timely manner and prolonging their time in the waiting area.

Healthcare systems and emergency departments have developed triage systems that best fit their specific needs. Great variations exist not only between different healthcare systems but even among EDs in the same country regarding the triage model adopted, personnel performing triage, and the triage process itself. Whatever triage system is chosen, it must meet the following requirements of being useful, valid, and reproducible. It must also be easy to use and classify, to help medical staff determine the acuity level in the shortest possible time [1,3].

The emergency department of Nikaia General Hospital, Nikaia, Greece is the busiest ED in Greece with more than 1000 ED visits in a 24 h shift. The emergency department of Larisa General Hospital, Greece has more than 300 ED visits in a 24 h shift. This overflow of incomings combined with other structural vulnerabilities of the Greek emergency healthcare system leads to prolonged waiting times from triage to seeing a physician with the right to treat, which in some cases may exceed 6 h. In 2018, we restructured our adult patient triage protocols, introducing a multi-layer triage approach based on the Swiss cheese model [4] (Figure 1). Our goal was to combine the strengths of accredited triage and early warning systems and scores to produce a process that would ensure that prolonged waiting times would not negatively impact patient outcomes [5].

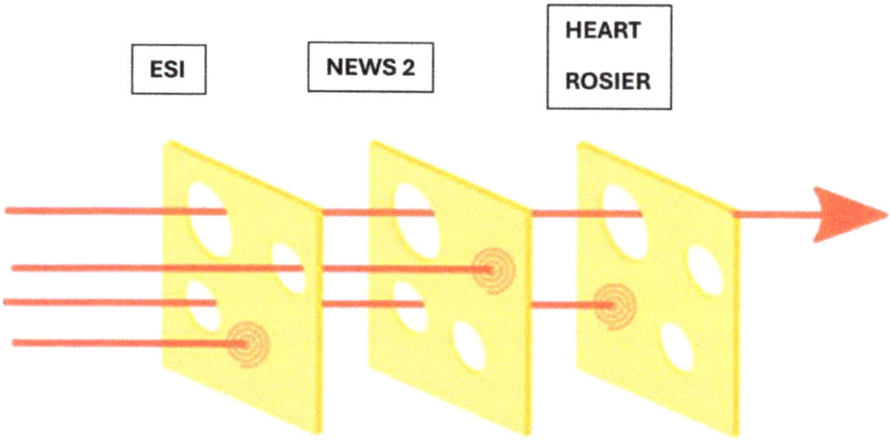

Figure 1. The multi-layer triage approach. Based on the Ben Aveling cheese model [6]. ESI, emergency severity index; NEWS 2, national early warning score 2.

Based on these principles, the Hellenic Society for Emergency Medicine developed a National Triage Proposal in 2024 [7].

2. Evaluating Existing Scoring Systems

Existing scoring systems can be roughly divided into three main categories.

2.1. Symptom-Based Triage Systems—Clinical Impression Triage Systems

The most widely used triage systems in this category are the Manchester triage system (MTS), the Australasian triage system (ATS), the emergency severity index (ESI), and the Canadian triage and acuity scale (CTAS). These 5-tier scoring systems are all well-validated and widely adopted in many EDs globally.

The outlines of each triage system are presented in Table 1.

There is still no clear advantage of one triage system over another [1,8,9].

Triage accuracy by all the above systems ranges between 56% and 87% [10]. All define very precisely and concordantly the highest (1 and 2) and the lowest (5) priorities while assigning priorities to the intermediate categories (3 and 4) was less precise for the adult population [1]. ESI has been reported to have a 20–30% under-tirage rate even for high acuity patients [11–16]. In our setting, when using ESI alone, accuracy was calculated at 63%, with an overall 23.6% under-triage rate [17]. Interpretation of vital sign deterioration has been identified as one of the factors leading to under-triage when using ESI [18].

Table 1. Characteristics of the most important five-level triage systems.

Parameter	ATS	MTS	CTAS	ESI
Time to initial assessment	10 min	ns	ns	ns
Time to contact with doctor with the right to treat	Immediate/10/60/ 120 min	Immediate/10/60/ 120/240 min	Immediate/15/30/ 60/120 min	Immediate/10 min/ ns
Re-triage	ns	As required	I:continuously; II: 15 min; III: 30 min; IV: 60 min; V: 120 min	As required
List of diagnoses or key symptoms	YES	52 key symptoms	YES	No
Training material	YES	YES	YES	YES

ATS, Australasian triage scale (previously national triage scale, NTS); CTAS, Canadian triage and acuity scale; MTS, Manchester triage scale; ESI, emergency severity index; ns, not specified; I to V: triage priority levels.

The strengths of symptom-based triage systems are that they are validated, fast, simple, and reliable for higher acuity patients (Priority 1 and Priority 2) and very low acuity patients (Priority 5). Their weaknesses include a high percentage of under-triage even for high acuity patients. They remain mainly subjective (depending on the level of training of the triage personnel) and thus not reproducible.

We chose to implement the ESI triage system mainly because there are no preset response times for each triage category and it fits better with our practice and policies so far. By choosing ESI almost 80% of our high acuity patients and our very low acuity patients should be identified quickly and accurately. A second triage layer would be needed to find these under-triaged critically ill patients and sort out medium and low-acuity patients. Since ESI is not symptom-based, we added several critical presenting symptom clusters from MTS, ATS, and CTAS as "Red Flag" symptoms to be recognized and prioritized accordingly.

2.2. Early Warning Scores (EWSs)

Early warning scores are based on the concept that altered physiology often precedes patient deterioration and death. Derangements in simple physiological observations (vital signs) can identify patients at high risk of deterioration. By recording and grading multiple parameters simultaneously, subtle changes in vital signs can be used to initiate early emergency management [19,20]. Most widespread are the rapid acute physiology score (RAPS), modified EWS (MEWS), modified EWS with Glasgow coma scale (GCS) (MEWS GCS), rapid emergency medicine score (REMS), Goodacre score, Worthing physiological score (WPS), Groarke score, VitalPac EWS (ViEWS), abbreviated VitalPac EWS (AbViEWS), Glasgow coma scale-age-systolic blood pressure score, vital sign score (VSS), National EWS (NEWS), and vital sign group (VSG) scores.

Early warning scores can accurately predict outcomes in several different populations [21,22]. They are excellent predictors of cardiac arrest, ICU transfer, and death in ICU, mortality within 2 days, deterioration within 2 days, and hospital admissions [21,23]. Among their advantages are accuracy, cross-specialty application, impact on communication, and opportunity for automation [23]. Their weak points are sensitivity, especially compared to specialty-specific scores, the need for practitioner engagement, and the need for clinical judgment.

EWSs have been proposed as emergency department triage tools [22]. EWS triage outperforms symptom-based triage in high-acuity patient recognition and risk stratification of mid-acuity patients [24].

There is no clear advantage to one EWS system over another [21]. We have chosen to integrate NEWS 2 into our multi-layer triage system. NEWS 2 is simple, easy to use, and reproducible. The vital signs are recorded on the table chart, and the score is calculated (Figure 2). Once the NEWS 2 score is calculated, appropriate response triggers are provided by the Royal College of Physicians (Figure 3) [25,26].

Physiological parameter	Score						
	3	2	1	0	1	2	3
Respiration rate (per minute)	≤8		9–11	12–20		21–24	≥25
SpO_2 Scale 1 (%)	≤91	92–93	94–95	≥96			
SpO_2 Scale 2 (%)	≤83	84–85	86–87	88–92 ≥93 on air	93–94 on oxygen	95–96 on oxygen	≥97 on oxygen
Air or oxygen?		Oxygen		Air			
Systolic blood pressure (mmHg)	≤90	91–100	101–110	111–219			≥220
Pulse (per minute)	≤40		41–50	51–90	91–110	111–130	≥131
Consciousness				Alert			CVPU
Temperature (°C)	≤35.0		35.1–36.0	36.1–38.0	38.1–39.0	≥39.1	

Figure 2. NEWS 2 chart. (Royal College of Physicians. National early warning score (NEWS) 2: standardizing the assessment of acute-illness severity in the NHS. Updated report of a working party. London: RCP, 2017).

NEW score	Clinical risk	Response
Aggregate score 0–4	Low	Ward-based response
Red score Score of 3 in any individual parameter	Low–medium	Urgent ward-based response*
Aggregate score 5–6	Medium	Key threshold for urgent response*
Aggregate score 7 or more	High	Urgent or emergency response**

* Response by a clinician or team with competence in the assessment and treatment of acutely ill patients and in recognising when the escalation of care to a critical care team is appropriate.

**The response team must also include staff with critical care skills, including airway management.

Figure 3. NEWS 2 thresholds and triggers. (Royal College of Physicians. National early warning score (NEWS) 2: standardizing the assessment of acute-illness severity in the NHS. Updated report of a working party. London: RCP, 2017).

Summarizing. NEWS 2 is a validated and easy-to-use score [27]. By choosing to add NEWS 2 as a second layer in our triage process, we address vital signs interpretation which was one of the most common error points in the triage systems mentioned above. We decrease the probability of under-triaging high acuity patients as NEWS 2 has better sensitivity in detecting high acuity patients that have been under-triaged in the previous step. By using the integrated thresholds and triggers, patients can subjectively and reproducibly be further triaged as middle and low acuity. Adding this layer slightly prolongs the triage process. This time delay will have a minimal impact on patient outcomes as the Priority 1 and Priority 2 patients who need immediate treatment have already been transferred to the treatment area by using ESI.

2.3. Specific Disease Scores

Time-sensitive, high mortality conditions might have atypical [28] or confusing presentations [29,30] on arrival, and minimal vital signs deterioration. Both acute coronary syndromes (ACSs) and stokes are among the leading causes of death and disability and early recognition and timely intervention are critical. As stated earlier, EWSs underperform compared to specialty-specific scores [31]. To detect these patients that have slipped through the first two triage layers, an extra layer is added consisting of disease-specific scores.

Many scores are in use to help identify patients with these conditions promptly and accurately. The most commonly used to detect ACS are the thrombosis in myocardial infarction risk (TIMI) score, the global registry of acute coronary events (GRACEs) score, and the HEART score. Likewise, the National institutes of health stroke scale (NIHSS), the Cincinnati prehospital stroke severity scale (CPSSS), the rapid arterial occlusion evaluation (RACE), the face arm speech test (FAST), the medic prehospital assessment for code stroke (MedPACS), and the recognition of stroke in the emergency room (ROSIER) are used for the early recognition of stroke.

The HEART score seems to perform better than other scores in detecting ACS [32,33]. In the mnemonic HEART, each letter corresponds to one of the following key pieces of the evaluation for patients with chest pain: history, ECG, age, risk factors, and troponin. Each component is scored on a scale of 0–2, with total scores ranging between 0 and 10 (Figure 4). The calculated score corresponds to the short-term probability of a major adverse cardiovascular event (MACE) and appropriate action is recommended [6] (Figure 5).

HEART Score

Element	Assessment	Points
History	Highly suspicious	2
	Moderately suspicious	1
	Slightly suspicious	0
Electrocardiogram	Significant ST depression	2
	Nonspecific repolarization disturbance	1
	Normal	0
Age	≥ 65 years	2
	45-65 years	1
	< 45 years	0
Risk factors	≥ 3 risk factors or history of atherosclerotic disease	2
	1 or 2 risk factors	1
	No risk factors known	0
Troponin	> 2x normal limit	2
	1-2x normal limit	1
	≤ normal limit	0

Figure 4. The HEART score [34].

Score	MACE	Mace over the next 6 weeks	Action
0–3	1.6%	2.5%	Early discharge
4–6	13%	20.3%	Clinical observation and non-invasive investigations
7–10	50%	72.2%	Early aggressive treatment

Figure 5. HEART score interpretation and stratification. (MACE = Major adverse cardiac events).

For detecting stroke in the emergency department, the ROSIER could be the test of choice as it has been well evaluated and showed consistently high sensitivity [35,36]. The ROSIER scale is a 7-item stroke recognition instrument employing clinical history and neurological signs, ranging from 2 to +5. A score of +1 or higher indicates a positive diagnosis of stroke or transient ischemic attack (TIA). The scale encompasses assessment criteria such as loss of consciousness, seizure activity, asymmetric facial, arm and leg weakness, speech disturbance, and visual field deficit (Figure 6).

Assessment Date ☐☐☐☐☐☐ Time ☐☐☐☐

Symptom onset Date ☐☐☐☐☐☐ Time ☐☐☐☐

GCS E=☐ M=☐ V=☐ **BP** ☐☐ ***BM** ☐

***If BM <3·5 mmol/L treat urgently and reassess once blood glucose normal**

Has there been loss of consciousness or syncope? Y (−1) ☐ N (0) ☐

Has there been seizure activity? Y (−1) ☐ N (0) ☐

Is there a NEW ACUTE onset (or on awakening from sleep)

I. Asymmetric facial weakness Y (+1) ☐ N (0) ☐

II. Asymmetric arm weakness Y (+1) ☐ N (0) ☐

III. Asymmetric leg weakness Y (+1) ☐ N (0) ☐

IV. Speech disturbance Y (+1) ☐ N (0) ☐

V. Visual field defect Y (+1) ☐ N (0) ☐

*Total Score ______ (−2 to +5)

Provisional diagnosis

☐Stroke ☐ Non-stroke (specify) ________________

*Stroke is unlikely but not completely excluded if total scores are ≤0.

Figure 6. Rosier scored [37]. BM, blood glucose; BP, blood pressure (mm Hg); GCS, Glasgow coma scale; E = eye; M = motor; V = verbal component.

Adding the ROSIER and HEART scores as an extra layer to our triage process minimizes the chance of under-triaging a life-threatening, time-sensitive disease. To perform these scores, certain blood tests are necessary. Blood glucose levels and troponin are essential parts of the algorithm. These create certain logistic needs (point care devices, blood sampling, personnel, etc.) that have a great impact on triage time. Depending on the setup, this might take from 10 to 30 min. In departments like ours with long waiting times, there is a clear benefit as under-triaged patients might lose their therapeutic window. The number of patients that end at this arm of our triage process is small and has minimal effect on the door-to-triage time for new incomings.

3. Proposing a Multilayer Triage System

Having an in-depth understanding of our emergency department's strengths and weaknesses and experience in conducting triage by ESI alone, we had identified areas of improvement of our triage process. Before introducing our institutional multilayer triage (Figure 7) system, an extensive and critical review of the literature was conducted. We combined the strong points of each score to better fit our needs. ESI would quickly and accurately identify the majority of very high acuity patients (Priority 1). ESI along with specific symptom clusters from ATS, MTS, and CTAS "Red flags" were used to identify quickly and accurately our high acuity patients (Priority 2). Acknowledging that almost 20% of Priority 1 and 2 patients might be under-triaged by ESI we introduced the NEWS 2 score as a second layer. In addition to increasing our Priority 1 and 2 detection rate, this addition also helped in a better interpretation of vital signs, and the objective and reproducible allocation of Priority 3 and Priority 4 patients. As an added benefit, it created an objective benchmark to which the patient's improvement or deterioration over time and response to treatment could be compared. ACS and stroke detection were a priority and a third layer consisting of the ROSIER and HEART scores was added allocating patients to Priority 2, 3, or 4. Those patients who at the end of the triage process were characterized as having low acuity were prioritized as Priority 4 or Priority 5 according to the estimated extent of investigation needed according to combined elements of the ESI (resources) and CTAS (age and comorbidities). Table 2 summarizes our priority allocation tools and scheme 1 depicts our triage process.

Table 2. Priority allocation summary.

Patient Priority	Clinical Condition	Tools Used to Identify
Priority 1	Immediate risk for life or limb	ESI
Priority 2	Serious enough or deteriorating so rapidly	ESI **and/or** Red Flags **and/or** NEWS 2 > 7 **and/or** HEART score >7 **and/or** Rosier > 1
Priority 3	Not serious enough, but could have atypical or early presentation of a serious condition	NEWS 2 = 5–6 **and/or** HEART score = 4–6
Priority 4	No serious underlying condition, but will require extensive work-up	ESI **and** NEWS 2 = 0–4 **and** HEART = 0–3 **and** Rosier ≤ 0
Priority 5	Acute but non-urgent or chronic problem without deterioration. Needs minimum investigation	ESI **and** NEWS 2 = 0–4 **and** HEART = 0–3 **and** Rosier < 0

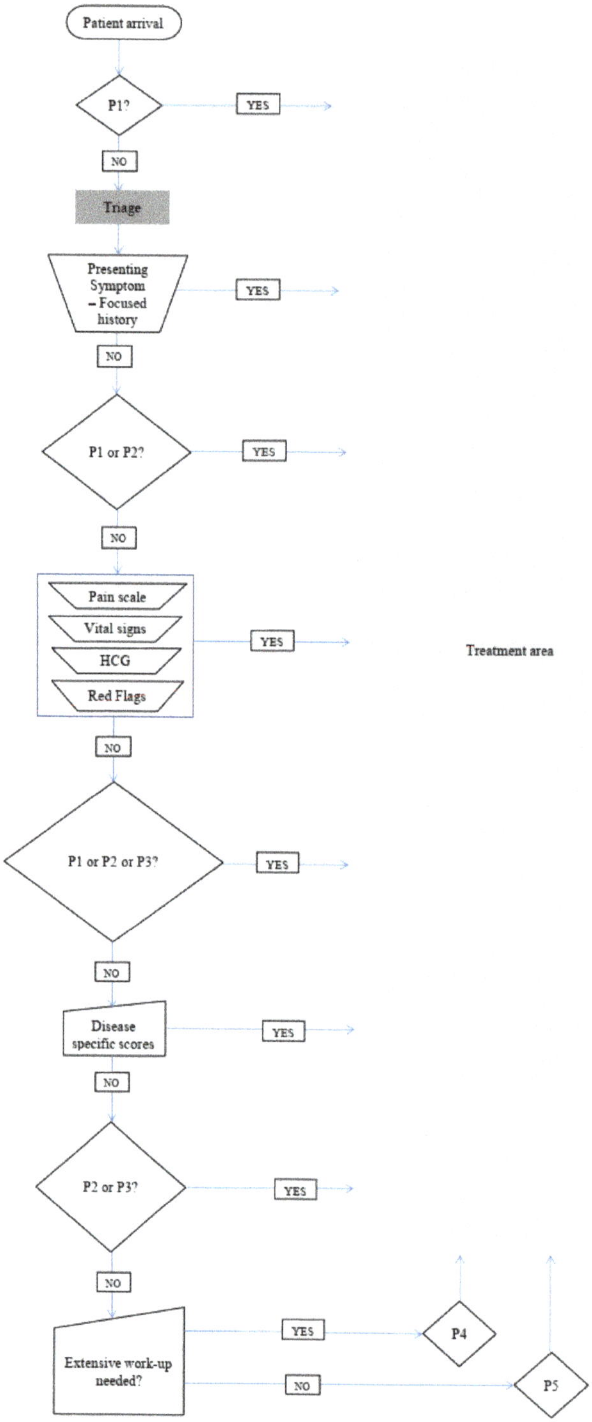

Figure 7. Scheme 1: the multilayer triage flow chart.

The steps of the multilayer triage system are as follows:

a. **Seeking Priority 1 patients**—Clinical impression.
   a. Use the basic principles of clinical impression triage systems such as ESI;
   b. "Is there an immediate risk for life or limb?";
   c. If the answer is YES, the patient is Priority 1;
   d. If the answer is NO, proceed to the next step.
b. **Seeking Priority 2 Patients**—Basic history taking and clinical impression.
   a. Use the basic principles of clinical impression triage systems such as ESI;
   b. "Is the patient's condition serious enough or deteriorating so rapidly that there is the potential of threat to life or organ system failure?";
   c. "Is the patient in severe pain?";
   d. "Does the patient have altered mental status?";
   e. "Are there any "Red Flags"?" CTAS, ATS, and MTS;
   f. If the answer is YES to any of the above questions, the Patient is Priority 2;
   g. If the answer is NO, proceed to the next step.
c. **Are you sure the Patient is NOT Priority 1 or 2?**—Vital signs.
   a. Use NEWS 2 to interpret vital signs;
   b. Prioritize the patient according to the EWS you have chosen;
      i. NEWS2 Score > 7: the patient is Priority 2;
      ii. NEWS2 Score 5–6 or a red score of 3 in any individual parameter: the patient is Priority 3
      iii. NEWS2 Score 0–4: proceed to the next step.
d. **Could the patient have an atypical presentation of a time-sensitive disease?**—Disease-specific scores.
   a. Use one of the accredited disease-specific scores depending on the clinical question;
   b. Prioritize the patient according to the score you have chosen;
   c. Use the HEART score for a possible ACS;
      i. For a HEART score of 7–10, the patient is Priority 2;
      ii. For a HEART score between 4 and 6, the patient is Priority 3;
      iii. For a HEART score of 0–3, proceed to the next step;
   d. Use the Rosier score for a possible stroke;
      i. For Rosier > 1, the patient is Priority 2;
      ii. For Rosier ≤ 0, proceed to the next step.
e. **Will this patient require extensive work-up?**—Focused history-taking.
   a. Use the basic principles of clinical impression triage systems such as ESI, and CTAS;
   b. "Will the patient, due to his age or comorbidities, require extensive work-up?";
   c. If the answer is YES, the patient is Priority 4;
   d. If the answer is NO, the Patient is Priority 5.

4. Results

Having implemented this multi-layer triage system for our adult population for more than 3 years, we have had almost no critical events in the waiting room. Few patients in the waiting room will need to change to a higher priority category while waiting. There is a very high level of agreement in the triage category between triage personnel of different training backgrounds. Although not systematically recorded, over-triage is below 15%. Our average triage time remains at 10 min. Even for the most complex arms of the chart, triage time never exceeds 25 min without prolonging our door-to-triage time. Our triage protocol has evolved over three years. A study protocol is running to evaluate its exact impact on triage accuracy and efficiency. A multi-center prospective study should be conducted to evaluate the effectiveness of this triage system in other EDs.

Having created an objective and reproducible system, training, reviewing, and quality control have become easier. Training triage healthcare personnel (ED medical doctors and nurses) is structured on our flowchart and the different scales used. Our training model consists of a 120 h theoretical course followed by 100 h supervised hands-on training. Monthly, our triage team critically reviews triage charts compared with patient outcomes and further didactic interventions are scheduled where needed.

More recently we have created and started implementing an artificial intelligence decision assistance tool built on these parameters. Artificial intelligence in triage has recently been a field of intensive research. Although the first reports seem very promising, there is still a lot to be undertaken until AI is widely available for ED triage [38,39].

Re-structuring the triage process alone has had multiple downstream effects with a positive impact on triage accuracy. A structured training program was implemented for triage personnel. Constant and systematic training of triage personnel has been shown to have a clear impact on triage quality. Our triage training program is being gradually adopted across Greece. Due to the new triage system, charting and recording had to be re-structured. Complete charting and strict adherence to the triage process have been identified as major contributors to high-quality triage. Re-triage at set time intervals was introduced as part of the quality control of the multilayer triage system. This created a re-triage culture that has remained. Even during our initial needs assessment and planning of the triage system, several ED throughput issues were identified and addressed accordingly.

5. Conclusions

Triage is the most vital part of ED operations and can have a great impact on ED flow and patient outcomes. The perfect triage system does not exist. Comparing different triage models is very difficult as this is a multi-factorial process depending on the input and output of patients, ED resources, staffing and hospital capabilities, training background of triage personnel, etc. Each emergency department must identify its own needs and tailor a triage process to fulfill them.

Author Contributions: Conceptualization of the model: D.T.; implementation: D.T., A.T. and D.B.; literature review: D.T. and D.B.; original draft preparation: D.T.; writing, reviewing, and editing: D.B. and A.T. All authors have read and agreed to the published version of the manuscript.

Funding: This research received no external funding.

Institutional Review Board Statement: Not applicable.

Informed Consent Statement: Not applicable.

Data Availability Statement: No new data were created or analyzed in this study.

Conflicts of Interest: The authors declare no conflicts of interest.

References

1. Ingielewicz, A.; Rychlik, P.; Sieminski, M. Drinking from the Holy Grail- Does a Perfect Triage System Exist? And Where to Look for It? J. *Pers. Med.* **2024**, *14*, 590. [CrossRef] [PubMed] [PubMed Central]
2. FitzGerald, G.; Jelinek, G.A.; Scott, D.; Gerdtz, M.F. Emergency department triage revisited. *Emerg. Med. J.* **2010**, *27*, 86–92. [CrossRef]

3. Alonso, P.S. Comparative analysis of global triage systems: Competencies of nursing and hospital and prehospital application. *J. Nurs. Valencia.* **2024**, 1–31.
4. Reason, J. *Managing the Risks of Organizational Accidents*, 1st ed.; Routledge: England, UK, 1997. [CrossRef]
5. Tsiftsis, D.; El-Fellah, N.; Dermatis, P. Systems and algorithms of Hospital Triage and patient Acuity Assessment in the Emer-gency Department. In *Intensive and Emergency Medicine: Scales, Algorithms, Protocols, Limits, Criteria and Indicators*, 22nd ed.; Baltopoulos, G., Ed.; Chapter in Greek; Ekdosis Epistimon: Athens, Attica Greece, 2019; pp. 301–309, ISBN 978-618-83535-5-8.
6. BenAveling—File: Swiss Cheese model.svg, CC BY-SA 4.0. Available online: https://commons.wikimedia.org/w/index.php?curid=133912327 (accessed on 3 March 2025).
7. Gatsouli, M.; Gerakari, S.; Ivkovitz, Z.; Intas, G.; Kalogridaki, M.; Karametos, I.; Lymperopoulou, D.; Pantazopoulos, I.; Paylidou, E.; Stavroulakis, S.; et al. Proposal of the Hellenic Society for Emergency Medicine for the Pilot Implementation of a National Triage System in Sites Providing Emergency Care Services. (Article in Greek). Available online: https://www.hesem.gr/%CF%80%CF%81%CF%8C%CF%84%CE%B1%CF%83%CE%B7-%CE%B5%CE%BB%CE%BB%CE%B7%CE%BD%CE%B9%CE%BA%CE%AE%CF%82-%CE%B5%CF%84%CE%B1%CE%B9%CF%81%CE%B5%CE%AF%CE%B1%CF%82-%CE%B5%CF%80%CE%B5%CE%AF%CE%B3%CE%BF%CF%85/ (accessed on 2 March 2025).
8. Kuriyama, A.; Urushidani, S.; Nakayama, T. Five-level emergency triage systems: Variation in assessment of validity. *Emerg. Med. J.* **2017**, *34*, 703–710. [CrossRef] [PubMed]
9. Christ, M.; Grossmann, F.; Winter, D.; Bingisser, R.; Platz, E. Modern triage in the emergency department. *Dtsch. Arztebl. Int.* **2010**, *107*, 892–898. [CrossRef] [PubMed] [PubMed Central]
10. Tam, H.L.; Chung, S.F.; Lou, C.K. A review of triage accuracy and future direction. *BMC Emerg. Med.* **2018**, *18*, 58. [CrossRef] [PubMed] [PubMed Central]
11. Storm-Versloot, M.N.; Ubbink, D.T.; Kappelhof, J.; Luitse, J.S. Comparison of an informally structured triage system, the emergency severity index, and the Manchester triage system to distinguish patient priority in the emergency department. *Acad. Emerg. Med.* **2011**, *18*, 822–829. [CrossRef] [PubMed]
12. Mistry, B.; Stewart De Ramirez, S.; Kelen, G.; Schmitz, P.S.K.; Balhara, K.S.; Levin, S.; Martinez, D.; Psoter, K.; Anton, X.; Hinson, J.S. Accuracy and Reliability of Emergency Department Triage Using the Emergency Severity Index: An International Multicenter Assessment. *Ann. Emerg. Med.* **2018**, *71*, 581–587.e3. [CrossRef] [PubMed]
13. Sax, D.R.; Warton, E.M.; Mark, D.G.; Vinson, D.R.; Kene, M.V.; Ballard, D.W.; Vitale, T.J.; McGaughey, K.R.; Beardsley, A.; Pines, J.M.; et al. Evaluation of the Emergency Severity Index in US Emergency Departments for the Rate of Mistriage. *JAMA Netw. Open* **2023**, *6*, e233404; Erratum in *JAMA Netw. Open* **2024**, *7*, e2423536. 10.1001/jamanetworkopen.2024.23536. [CrossRef] [PubMed] [PubMed Central]
14. Zachariasse, J.M.; van der Hagen, V.; Seiger, N.; Mackway-Jones, K.; van Veen, M.; Moll, H.A. Performance of triage systems in emergency care: A systematic review and meta-analysis. *BMJ Open* **2019**, *9*, e026471. [CrossRef] [PubMed] [PubMed Central]
15. Suamchaiyaphum, K.; Jones, A.R.; Polancich, S. The accuracy of triage classification using Emergency Severity Index. *Int. Emerg. Nurs.* **2024**, *77*, 101537. [CrossRef] [PubMed]
16. Peta, D.; Day, A.; Lugari, W.S.; Gorman, V.; Ahayalimudin, N.; Pajo, V.M.T. Triage: A Global Perspective. *J. Emerg. Nurs.* **2023**, *49*, 814–825. [CrossRef] [PubMed]
17. El-Fellah, N.; Dritsa, A.; Dermatis, P.; Intas, G.; Papadopoulos, G.; Kaklamanou, E.; Tsiftsis, D. Knowledge of Health Care Professionals of the Emergency Department of the Hospital of N. Attica in the Emergency Severity Index Triage System. *Hell. J. Nurs.* **2017**, *56*, 358–365. (In Greek)
18. Rashid, K.; Ullah, M.; Ahmed, S.T.; Sajid, M.Z.; Hayat, M.A.; Nawaz, B.; Abbas, K. Accuracy of Emergency Room Triage Using Emergency Severity Index (ESI): Independent Predictor of Under and Over Triage. *Cureus* **2021**, *13*, e20229. [CrossRef] [PubMed] [PubMed Central]
19. Goldhill, D.R.; McNarry, A.F. Physiological abnormalities in early warning scores are related to mortality in adult inpatients. *Br. J. Anaesth.* **2004**, *92*, 882–884. [CrossRef] [PubMed]
20. Ridley, S. The recognition and early management of critical illness. *Ann. R. Coll. Surg. Engl.* **2005**, *87*, 315–322. [CrossRef]
21. Spencer, W.; Smith, J.; Date, P.; de Tonnerre, E.; Taylor, D.M. Determination of the best early warning scores to predict clinical outcomes of patients in the emergency department. *Emerg. Med. J.* **2019**, *36*, 716–721. [CrossRef] [PubMed]
22. Kramer, A.A.; Sebat, F.; Lissauer, M. A review of early warning systems for prompt detection of patients at risk for clinical decline. *J. Trauma. Acute Care Surg.* **2019**, *87* (Suppl. S1), S67–S73. [CrossRef] [PubMed]
23. Downey, C.L.; Tahir, W.; Randell, R.; Brown, J.M.; Jayne, D.G. Strengths and limitations of early warning scores: A systematic review and narrative synthesis. *Int. J. Nurs. Stud.* **2017**, *76*, 106–119. [CrossRef] [PubMed]
24. Schinkel, M.; Bergsma, L.; Veldhuis, L.I.; Ridderikhof, M.L.; Holleman, F. Comparing complaint-based triage scales and early warning scores for emergency department triage. *Emerg. Med. J.* **2022**, *39*, 691–696. [CrossRef] [PubMed] [PubMed Central]
25. Williams, B. The National Early Warning Score: From concept to NHS implementation. *Clin. Med.* **2022**, *22*, 499–505. [CrossRef] [PubMed] [PubMed Central]

26. Royal College of Physicians. *National Early Warning Score (NEWS) 2: Standardising the Assessment of Acute-Illness Severity in the NHS. Updated Report of a Working Party*; RCP: London, UK, 2017.
27. Smith, G.B.; Prytherch, D.R.; Meredith, P.; Schmidt, P.E.; Featherstone, P.I. The ability of the National Early Warning Score (NEWS) to discriminate patients at risk of early cardiac arrest, unanticipated intensive care unit admission, and death. *Resuscitation* **2013**, *84*, 465–470. [CrossRef] [PubMed]
28. Khan, I.A.; Karim, H.M.R.; Panda, C.K.; Ahmed, G.; Nayak, S. Atypical Presentations of Myocardial Infarction: A Systematic Review of Case Reports. *Cureus* **2023**, *15*, e35492. [CrossRef] [PubMed] [PubMed Central]
29. Vilela, P. Acute stroke differential diagnosis: Stroke mimics. *Eur. J. Radiol.* **2017**, *96*, 133–144. [CrossRef] [PubMed]
30. Pohl, M.; Hesszenberger, D.; Kapus, K.; Meszaros, J.; Feher, A.; Varadi, I.; Pusch, G.; Fejes, E.; Tibold, A.; Feher, G. Ischemic stroke mimics: A comprehensive review. *J. Clin. Neurosci.* **2021**, *93*, 174–182. [CrossRef] [PubMed]
31. Nishi, F.A.; de Oliveira Motta Maia, F.; de Souza Santos, I.; de Almeida Lopes Monteiro da Cruz, D. Assessing sensitivity and specificity of the Manchester Triage System in the evaluation of acute coronary syndrome in adult patients in emergency care: A systematic review. *JBI Database Syst. Rev. Implement. Rep.* **2017**, *15*, 1747–1761. [CrossRef] [PubMed]
32. Ashburn, N.P.; O'Neill, J.C.; Stopyra, J.P.; Mahler, S.A. Scoring systems for the triage and assessment of short-term cardiovascular risk in patients with acute chest pain. *Rev. Cardiovasc. Med.* **2021**, *22*, 1393–1403. [CrossRef] [PubMed] [PubMed Central]
33. Ke, J.; Chen, Y.; Wang, X.; Wu, Z.; Chen, F. Indirect comparison of TIMI, HEART, and GRACE for predicting major cardiovascular events in patients admitted to the emergency department with acute chest pain: A systematic review and meta-analysis. *BMJ Open* **2021**, *11*, e048356. [CrossRef] [PubMed] [PubMed Central]
34. Aung, S.S.M.; Roongsritong, C. A Closer Look at the HEART Score. *Cardiol. Res.* **2022**, *13*, 255–263. [CrossRef] [PubMed] [PubMed Central]
35. Zhelev, Z.; Walker, G.; Henschke, N.; Fridhandler, J.; Yip, S. Prehospital stroke scales as screening tools for early identification of stroke and transient ischemic attack. *Cochrane Database Syst. Rev.* **2019**, *4*, CD011427. [CrossRef] [PubMed] [PubMed Central]
36. Chehregani Rad, I.; Azimi, A. Recognition of Stroke in the Emergency Room (ROSIER) Scale in Identifying Strokes and Transient Ischemic Attacks (TIAs); a Systematic Review and Meta-Analysis. *Arch. Acad. Emerg. Med.* **2023**, *11*, e67. [CrossRef] [PubMed] [PubMed Central]
37. Nor, A.M.; Davis, J.; Sen, B.; Shipsey, D.; Louw, S.J.; Dyker, A.G.; Davis, M.; Ford, G.A. The Recognition of Stroke in the Emergency Room (ROSIER) scale: Development and validation of a stroke recognition instrument. *Lancet Neurol.* **2005**, *4*, 727–734. [CrossRef] [PubMed]
38. Tyler, S.; Olis, M.; Aust, N.; Patel, L.; Simon, L.; Triantafyllidis, C.; Patel, V.; Lee, D.W.; Ginsberg, B.; Ahmad, H.; et al. Use of Artificial Intelligence in Triage in Hospital Emergency Departments: A Scoping Review. *Cureus* **2024**, *16*, e59906. [CrossRef] [PubMed] [PubMed Central]
39. Piliuk, K.; Tomforde, S. Artificial intelligence in emergency medicine. A systematic literature review. *Int. J. Med. Inform.* **2023**, *180*, 105274. [CrossRef] [PubMed]

healthcare

MDPI

Systematic Review

Uterotonic Drugs in Prevention and Management in Postpartum Haemorrhage in Prehospital Deliveries—A Systematic Review

Hanna Wiciak [1], Mateusz Strózik [2] and Jacek Smereka [3,*]

1 Clinical Department of Gynecologic Surgery and Oncology, University Center of Obstetrics and Gynecology, Wroclaw Medical University, 50-367 Wroclaw, Poland; hanna.wiciak@umw.edu.pl
2 Clinical Department of Obstetrics and Gynecology, University Center of Obstetrics and Gynecology, Wroclaw Medical University, 50-367 Wroclaw, Poland; m.strozik@umw.edu.pl
3 Department of Emergency Medical Service, Wroclaw Medical University, 50-367 Wroclaw, Poland
* Correspondence: jacek.smereka@umw.edu.pl

Abstract: Background: Obstetric haemorrhage, particularly postpartum haemorrhage (PPH), remains a significant global health challenge and a leading cause of maternal mortality. Despite advancements in understanding and preventing PPH, haemorrhage remains a leading cause of maternal mortality worldwide. The aim of this study was to review the current literature on the use of uterotonic drugs, particularly oxytocin, in reducing perinatal mortality during prehospital deliveries. Methods: In December 2024, a comprehensive search was conducted across PubMed, Web of Science, Embase, and Scopus, yielding 108 records, of which four studies met the inclusion criteria. Results: The limited evidence underscores the need for targeted research and adherence to international obstetric guidelines to improve PPH management and maternal outcomes. In some countries, the only uterotonic drug available in all EMS teams is oxytocin; in others, there is none. Emergency Medical Services (EMS) play a critical role in providing lifesaving interventions during obstetric emergencies, often serving as the first and sometimes only point of medical contact for women experiencing complications during childbirth. Conclusion: There is a lack of high-quality clinical studies evaluating the effectiveness of uterotonic agents in EMS operations and their role in treating postpartum haemorrhage in prehospital settings. Addressing this gap requires targeted research to generate robust evidence and inform the development of standardized protocols. Such efforts could enhance the timely management of PPH, ultimately reducing maternal mortality and improving outcomes in resource-limited and prehospital environments. By bridging the evidence gap, EMS systems worldwide can be better equipped to handle obstetric emergencies effectively.

Keywords: ambulance; paramedic; prehospital delivery; postpartum haemorrhage; oxytocin; uterotonic drugs

1. Introduction

Obstetric haemorrhage, particularly postpartum haemorrhage (PPH), remains a significant global health challenge and a leading cause of maternal mortality. Despite advancements in understanding and preventing PPH, haemorrhage remains a leading cause of maternal mortality worldwide. According to a systematic analysis, haemorrhage was responsible for 34% of the 275,000 estimated global maternal deaths in 2015, highlighting the critical need for sustained efforts to improve prevention, management, and access to effective interventions, particularly in resource-limited settings [1].

Although the definitions of postpartum haemorrhage vary among scientific organizations—the World Health Organization (WHO) [2] defines it as blood loss of >500 mL within 24 h of childbirth, the American College of Obstetricians and Gynecologists (ACOG) [3] as >1000 mL within the same timeframe, and the Society of Obstetricians and Gynaecologists (SOGC) [4] as any blood loss that threatens haemodynamic stability—research published to date indicates that the uterotonic is the most important component in preventing PPH [5]. Despite these definitional differences, research consistently identifies uterotonic agents—especially oxytocin—as the cornerstone of PPH prevention.

While previous systematic reviews, such as De Silva's, have explored PPH management in hospital settings, limited attention has been given to prehospital care, where Emergency Medical Services (EMS) often provide the first and sometimes only medical intervention [6]. Given the variability in EMS protocols and the availability of uterotonic drugs, a focused review of their role in prehospital settings is necessary. This study aims to evaluate the existing literature on the use of uterotonic drugs by EMS in managing PPH, identifying gaps in knowledge and areas for improvement.

2. Material and Methods

2.1. Study Design

This systematic review was conducted in adherence to the PRISMA (Preferred Reporting Items for Systematic Reviews and Meta-Analyses) guidelines to ensure methodological transparency and consistency in the analysis process. The PICO framework (Population, Intervention, Comparison, Outcome) was used to define the research question and guide the selection process.

2.2. Research Question

Using the PICO model, the research question was defined as follows: What is the impact of uterotonic drug administration in a prehospital setting on perinatal outcomes, particularly in the context of deliveries managed by Emergency Medical Services (EMS)?

- Population (P): Women giving birth in prehospital settings, specifically deliveries occurring outside hospital facilities and attended by emergency medical services (EMS) teams.
- Intervention (I): Administration of uterotonic drugs (e.g., oxytocin, carbetocin, misoprostol, ergometrine) to prevent or manage obstetric complications such as postpartum haemorrhage.
- Comparison (C): No uterotonic treatment or alternative management strategies.
- Outcome (O): Perinatal outcomes (including maternal and neonatal mortality) and other clinical outcomes, such as postpartum haemorrhage, neonatal complications, and adverse events related to uterotonic use.

The PICO framework guided the search strategy development and the selection criteria for eligible studies, ensuring that the review systematically addressed the impact of uterotonic drugs in prehospital obstetric care.

2.3. Search Strategy

A comprehensive database search was concluded in December 2024 using four electronic databases—PubMed, Web of Science, Embase, and Scopus—to identify articles addressing the central research question. The search strategy involved combining terms related to the following:

- Uterotonic agents: "uterotonic drugs", "oxytocin", "misoprostol", "ergometrine", and "carbetocin";
- Prehospital obstetric care: "prehospital delivery", "out-of-hospital birth", "emergency obstetric care", "paramedics", "ambulance", and "EMS obstetric care";
- Outcomes: "perinatal mortality", "maternal mortality", and "neonatal outcomes".

Search terms were adjusted for each database's indexing system. No publication date limits were applied. Only articles published in English were included.

2.4. Eligibility Criteria

Inclusion Criteria:

- Studies involving the administration of uterotonic agents in prehospital childbirth attended by EMS;
- Clinical trials, observational studies, or systemic reviews with extractable data;
- Studies reporting on maternal or neonatal outcomes.

Exclusion criteria:

- Studies conducted exclusively in hospital settings;
- Case reports, editorials, opinion pieces, and letters without original data;
- Articles not available in full-text or not in English.

Rationale:

Due to the limited number of studies available on prehospital PPH management, broad inclusion criteria were used to maximize the scope of evidence while maintaining relevance to the research question.

2.5. Study Selection

A total of 108 articles were identified across all databases. After eliminating 41 duplicates, 67 unique articles remained. Titles and abstracts were screened for relevance by two independent reviewers. Full-text review was conducted for eligible articles, resulting in 4 studies included in the final analysis.

2.6. Data Extraction

Data were extracted independently by two reviewers into a structured table capturing the following:

- Study design and setting;
- Population characteristics;
- Type of uterotonic used;
- EMS protocols or procedures;
- Reported outcomes (e.g., maternal mortality, PPH rates, adverse events).

Disagreements were resolved through discussion.

2.7. Quality Assessment

Due to the small number of included studies, a formal risk of bias assessment was not feasible. However, methodological quality was considered during narrative synthesis, and limitations were acknowledged in the discussion.

2.8. Data Synthesis

Given the heterogeneity in study design, outcome reporting, and intervention specifics, a narrative synthesis approach was adopted instead of a meta-analysis. Key findings were summarized descriptively and compared thematically.

2.9. Flow Diagram

A Reporting Items for Systematic Review and Meta-analysis (PRISMA) flow diagram was utilized to visually present the study selection process (Figure 1).

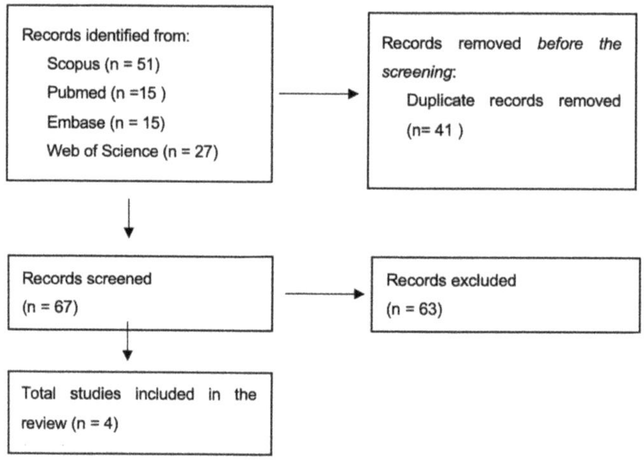

Figure 1. PRISMA flow diagram showing study selection.

3. Results

3.1. Study Characteristics

A total of four studies met the inclusion criteria for this review. These included one systematic review and three retrospective observational studies published between 2020 and 2024. Sample sizes ranged from 62 to 350 participants or cases. All studies focused on using oxytocin in prehospital or out-of-hospital (OOH) obstetric care provided by Emergency Medical Services (EMS). The included studies were conducted in different geographical regions and varied in terms of protocols, population, and specific outcomes assessed (Table 1).

Table 1. Studies addressing the impact of uterotonic drugs in prehospital obstetric care.

Author, Year	Sample Size	Aim	Participant Characteristics	Study Design	Main Results	Newcastle–Ottawa Quality Score
De Silva et al., 2022 [6]	6 studies included in the review	To determine the efficacy of pharmacological management: oxytocin, compared to TXA, in women suffering PPH in the out-of-hospital environment.	Studies including women with PPH in rural or out-of-hospital settings.	Systematic review	In the out-of-hospital setting, there is no difference in blood loss, neonatal or maternal mortality, morbidity, or need for further interventions when using oxytocin compared to no intervention or standard care for PPH.	8

Table 1. *Cont.*

Author, Year	Sample Size	Aim	Participant Characteristics	Study Design	Main Results	Newcastle–Ottawa Quality Score
Wiciak et al., 2024 [7]	62 real situations when paramedics used oxytocin	To assess the rate of oxytocin use by paramedics during out-of-hospital births.	Women delivering outside of hospital settings in Poland; retrospective data from EMS services.	Retrospective observational study.	Polish EMS teams rarely administer oxytocin at the prehospital stage.	6
Schultz et al., 2021 [8]	350 OOH births were included in this study	Describes the prehospital administration of oxytocin by paramedics following attendance of out-of-hospital (OOH) births.	Retrospective review of EMS data.	Retrospective observational study.	Oxytocin is a well-accepted and safe treatment adjunct for the management of the third stage of labour in OOH births. It should be considered for routine practice by other emergency medical services.	5
E Klemettilä et al., 2020 [9]	216 analysed out-of-hospital deliveries	To determine whether the use of oxytocin is associated with diminished postpartum haemorrhage after unplanned out-of-hospital deliveries.	Women with unplanned out-of-hospital deliveries treated by EMS.	Retrospective and non-randomized.	Oxytocin administered by ambulance personnel after an unplanned out-of-hospital delivery was not associated with diminished PPH.	6

3.2. Interventions and Outcomes

Across all studies, oxytocin was the main uterotonic agent investigated. The systematic review by De Silva et al. compared oxytocin with tranexamic acid (TXA) and concluded that in the out-of-hospital environment, there were no significant differences in blood loss, maternal or neonatal morbidity, or need for further interventions between oxytocin and standard care. This study represented the most comprehensive approach but included a broader definition of "out of hospital", encompassing rural and low-resource environments [6].

The observational studies focused primarily on oxytocin's real-world use and outcomes in EMS contexts. Wiciak et al. analysed EMS records from Poland and found that paramedics rarely administrated oxytocin despite its inclusion in national protocols [7]. Schultz et al. described oxytocin as a well-accepted and safe addition in management during the third stage of labour, suggesting that the EMS system should consider using it as a routine [8]. However, Klemettilä et al. reported no significant association between oxytocin use and a reduction in PPH, raising questions about its clinical effectiveness when administered late or under uncontrolled prehospital conditions [9].

3.3. Quality Assessment

The Newcastle–Ottawa Scale (NOS) guided the evaluation of the methodological quality of the included studies. The systematic review by De Silva scored 8 out of 9 points, reflecting a strong methodological design, robust inclusion criteria, and use of comparative groups. The three observational studies (Klemettilä, Schultz, Wiciak) [7–9] scored between 5 and 6 points, mainly due to limitations such as the absence of randomization, control groups, and follow-up data. Despite these limitations, they provided significant contextual evidence regarding the feasibility and safety of uterotonic use in EMS practice.

3.4. Comparison with Existing Literature

The discrepancy between the number of studies included in this review ($n = 4$) and those reported in De Silva's review ($n = 6$) can be attributed to differences in inclusion criteria and review focus. While De Silva et al. examined a broader range of interventions (e.g., including TXA) and settings (including rural, but not strictly EMS-attended births), the present review applied narrower eligibility criteria emphasizing prehospital obstetric care conducted by EMS personnel and specifically the administration of uterotonics like oxytocin [6]. This narrower scope strengthens the specificity and relevance of the findings to EMS systems but also highlights the limited volume of high-quality research available on this topic.

4. Discussion

The management of postpartum haemorrhage (PPH) in out-of-hospital deliveries remains a unique challenge for emergency medical services (EMS) worldwide. Our review points out critical gaps in prehospital care, including variability in uterotonic drug use, limited EMS protocols, and significant logistical barriers. While oxytocin continues to be a cornerstone of PPH prevention in clinical settings, its role in the emergency context is still uncertain and underexplored.

4.1. Prehospital Deliveries

Prehospital birth refers to a situation known as birth before arrival or an unplanned out-of-hospital delivery during which a newborn is delivered unexpectedly outside of a hospital setting. This is a highly challenging and exceptional situation, as these events occur suddenly in places that lack proper equipment and often do not have adequately trained or experienced personnel on-site [10]. Out-of-hospital (OOH) emergency deliveries are often viewed by emergency medical service (EMS) providers as either a uniquely joyful experience or one of the most daunting and challenging moments of their careers [11,12].

Prehospital deliveries are associated with certain risks of complications and unpredictable courses resulting from various factors. First and foremost, the issue of proper qualification for a home birth conducted in an elective setting, often with the participation of a midwife, is important. In some countries, the percentage of these births is relatively high. In the Netherlands, the percentage of home births was 16.3% in both 2015 and 2019. In comparison, other countries reported much lower rates: 1.4% in Denmark, 1.3% in Germany, 1.1% in Belgium, 0.9% in Hungary, 0.32% in Spain, 0.2% in Finland, and 0.03% in Poland [13]. Another issue is that emergency deliveries are not initially planned as home deliveries, including deliveries attended by EMS team personnel [14]. The EMS teams' staff, physicians, nurses, and paramedics are properly trained to assist patients during out-of-hospital deliveries, including treating complications associated with childbirth and caring for the newborn [15]. There are significant gaps in the training of EMS teams, particularly in managing postpartum haemorrhage. Additionally, there are issues with the documentation process, which is often incomplete and lacks important details, including an assessment of the severity of PPH [16].

A critical issue is the ability of EMS teams to assist with postpartum haemorrhage, including the availability of appropriate medications in the ambulance and transparent procedures for their use [17]. In many countries, oxytocin and other similarly acting drugs are not standard in EMS ambulances, while paramedics are not allowed to administer the drug without a physician's order [8,18].

Another crucial aspect of unplanned out-of-hospital delivery is the poorer outcomes for the newborn. Currently, there is no doubt that these deliveries are associated with an increased risk of perinatal mortality and neonatal morbidity, regardless of the gestational age. Several studies highlight the important role of the EMS call handler in providing essential guidance during prehospital deliveries. Key themes identified in the call-handler advice include the following: (1) the importance of neonatal temperature, (2) where to place the baby after birth, (3) methods to keep the baby warm, (4) the timing of temperature management, and (5) the clarity and priority of instructions. Proper training of EMS teams can significantly improve perinatal outcomes in prehospital settings [19–22].

From the perspective of emergency medical care, it is essential to note that prolonged transportation time is a significant predictor of neonatal mortality. Additionally, neonatal interventions before and during transport significantly impact neonatal morbidity and mortality [23–25].

Since paramedics most often assist BBA patients, adequate training (including practical skills) is essential to effectively care for them during this period. Paramedics must build confidence in their ability to support the newborn's adjustment to the extra-uterine environment and ensure that the third stage of labour progresses without complications for the mother. Furthermore, ideally, they should possess the clinical skills to respond promptly to any complications that may arise.

An issue of importance is the potential cooperation of paramedics and midwives at the prehospital stage, including, in particular, the education of paramedics in assisting with out-of-hospital deliveries [26].

4.2. Novelty and Aim

To our knowledge, this is the first systematic review focused specifically on the use of uterotonic agents—particularly oxytocin—by emergency medical services (EMS) teams during out-of-hospital deliveries. While active management of the third stage of labour is widely recognized in obstetric care, its implementation in emergency and out-of-hospital settings remains underexplored.

4.3. Interpretation of Findings

The studies reviewed report that oxytocin administration in prehospital deliveries is inconsistent and often very restricted. Schultz et al. [8] showed relatively frequent administration of oxytocin in Australia (63.4%), while in Finland [9] and Poland [7], oxytocin use was markedly lower due to logistical and regulatory limitations. Notably, none of the included studies proved a significant decrease in the incidence or severity of postpartum haemorrhage (PPH) associated with prehospital oxytocin use. While safety was generally affirmed, the lack of a consistent benefit suggests other factors—such as timing, route of administration, and staff training—may affect outcomes.

4.4. International Guidelines and Recommendations

The recommendations from the main scientific organizations that issue guidelines for the management of postpartum haemorrhage, such as ACOG (American College of Obstetricians and Gynecologists), RCOG (Royal College of Obstetricians and Gynaecologists), FIGO (International Federation of Gynecology and Obstetrics), RANZCOG (Royal Australian and New Zealand College of Obstetricians and Gynaecologists), SOGC (Society of Obstetricians and Gynaecologists of Canada), and the WHO (World Health Organization), despite variations, are consistent in highlighting the importance of the active management of the third stage of labour for preventing postpartum haemorrhage. They recommend several interventions, with oxytocin being the standard criterion [27–31]. The European Society of Anaesthesiology and Intensive Care emphasizes the critical need for rapid intervention to prevent and manage postpartum haemorrhage. Quick action significantly improves the chances of therapeutic success. Furthermore, when possible in prehospital settings, 1 g of tranexamic acid is recommended, as it can aid in controlling the haemorrhage [32]. The collected and summarized recommendations for treating PPH are presented in Table 2. The authors did not find direct guidelines regarding EMS and perinatal care. The absence of unified, enforceable protocols in EMS systems undermines the consistent application of these evidence-based recommendations in out-of-hospital environments. The value of adopting globally endorsed protocols cannot be overstated: they provide clarity, support clinical decision-making under pressure, and ensure that all in-labour patients—regardless of setting—receive a minimum standard of care. Inconsistencies in drug availability and administration authority between regions or services risk preventable maternal morbidity and mortality.

Table 2. Comparison of recommendations from different organizations for the treatment of PPH.

Aspect	The Primary Cause of PPH Recognized as	First-Line Uterotonic Drug	Second-Line Uterotonic Agent	Adjunct Therapy	Timing of TXA
WHO	Uterine atony	Oxytocin 10 IU IM/IV. IV infusion of 10–40 IU in 1000 mL isotonic crystalloids flow. Maximum dose not specified.	Ergometrine 0.2 mg IM/IV (if no hypertension and/or preeclampsia). Misoprostol 800 µg sublingual (if oxytocin is unavailable). Carboprost 250 µg IM (if no asthma).	Tranexamic Acid (TXA) 1 g IV within 3 h of birth.	Administer as soon as possible, within 3 h of PPH onset.
FIGO	Uterine atony	Oxytocin 10 IU IM/IV. IV infusion of 10–40 IU in 1000 mL isotonic crystalloids at 100–200 mL/h flow. Maximum dose not specified.	Misoprostol 800 µg sublingual or rectal. Ergometrine 0.2 mg IM/IV (if no hypertension and/or preeclampsia). Carboprost 250 µg IM (if no asthma).	Tranexamic Acid (TXA) 1 g IV in cases of trauma or coagulopathy.	Administer as early as possible.
RCOG	Uterine atony	Oxytocin 5 IU IV slow bolus or 10 IU IM. IV infusion of 40 IU in 500 mL isotonic crystalloids at 125 mL/h flow. The maximum dose for IV infusion is 40 IU.	Ergometrine 0.5 mg slowly IV/IM (if no hypertension and/or preeclampsia). Carboprost 250 µg IM. repeated at intervals of not less than 15 min to a maximum of eight doses (if no asthma). Misoprostol 600 µg orally or 800 µg rectally.	Tranexamic Acid (TXA) 1 g IV, repeat if needed after 30 min.	Administer as soon as possible, within 3 h of onset.
ACOG	Uterine atony	Oxytocin 10–40 IU IV infusion or 10 IU IM. IV infusion of 10–40 IU in 1000 mL isotonic crystalloids. The maximum dose for IV infusion is 40 IU.	Methylergonovine 0.2 mg IM. Carboprost 250 µg IM (if no asthma). Misoprostol 800–1000 µg rectally.	Tranexamic Acid (TXA) 1 g IV, may repeat after 30 min.	Administer within 3 h of PPH onset.

Table 2. *Cont.*

Aspect	The Primary Cause of PPH Recognized as	First-Line Uterotonic Drug	Second-Line Uterotonic Agent	Adjunct Therapy	Timing of TXA
SOGC	Uterine atony	Oxytocin 10 IU IM or 20–40 IU IV infusion. IV infusion of 10–40 IU in 1000 mL isotonic crystalloids at 125 mL/hour flow.	Ergometrine 0.2 mg slowly (over 60 s) IM/IV (if no hypertension and/or preeclampsia). Carboprost 250 µg IM (if no asthma). Misoprostol 600–1000 µg rectally or orally.	Tranexamic Acid (TXA) 1 g IV, repeat after 30 min if needed.	Administer within 3 h of PPH onset.
RANZCOG	Uterine atony	Oxytocin Initial 5 IU IV slow bolus 10 IU IM/IV. IV infusion of 10–40 IU in 1000 mL isotonic crystalloids. The maximum dose for IV infusion is 40 IU.	Misoprostol 800–1000 µg rectally or sublingually. Carboprost 250 µg IM repeated at intervals of not less than 15 min to a maximum of eight doses (if no asthma).	Tranexamic Acid (TXA) 1 g IV, repeat if needed after 30 min.	Administer within 3 h of PPH onset.

4.5. *Uterotonic Drugs in Prehospital Deliveries Attended by EMS Teams*

After reviewing the literature, only a few articles on the use of uterotonic drugs in prehospital deliveries involving EMS personnel were found.

A study published by Schultz et al. in 2021 retrospectively analysed all out-of-hospital deliveries in 2018 attended by Queensland Ambulance Service teams in Australia. Of 350 out-of-hospital deliveries, oxytocin was administered in 222 cases (63.4%). In contrast, in 19.1% of cases, patients refused oxytocin administration, and in 17.4% of cases, the paramedic decided not to administer oxytocin. There were no cases of complications or side effects associated with the administration of oxytocin, which was, on average, administered 14 min after the birth of the child [8].

Klemettilä et al. performed a retrospective analysis of out-of-hospital deliveries in the area covered by Helsinki University Hospital in Finland over 5 years from 2013 to 2017. The authors found that oxytocin was available in ambulances serving half of the study population while not in the rest. During the study period, 216 out-of-hospital deliveries were found, with oxytocin available in ambulances in 111 cases. In half of these cases (57 of the 111 deliveries), oxytocin was administered. However, there was no difference in the severity of postpartum haemorrhage compared to cases in which oxytocin was not given. The study's conclusions suggested that oxytocin is not essential in emergency team settings [9].

Wiciak et al. analysed cases of oxytocin administration between 2018 and 2023 in Poland. The authors showed that EMS teams used oxytocin in only 62 out-of-hospital deliveries, representing less than 7% of all 879 deliveries in this period in which EMS teams in Poland were involved. The percentage of oxytocin use is very low due to its availability in ambulances and the ability of paramedics to administer it [7].

The authors' opinion is that the results of our systematic review are highly surprising, and contrary to the expected results. Our study revealed no significant reduction in postpartum haemorrhage despite widespread oxytocin in labour rooms. The lack of comprehensive studies, the absence of unified administration protocols, and potential delays or imprecise drug delivery in prehospital environments significantly challenge the systematic evaluation of oxytocin's effectiveness in out-of-hospital settings.

Several factors may explain why oxytocin has not significantly reduced blood loss in the prehospital setting. Delays in drug administration due to post-delivery logistics, managing a newborn as another patient for the same team, or transport priorities may reduce its effectiveness. Medication routes of administration might play a role: intramuscular administration—more common in an out-of-hospital environment—may have a slower onset than intravenous administration.

Although EMS teams are usually equipped to monitor vital signs, continuous or comprehensive maternal monitoring—such as accurate blood loss estimation and uterine assessment—is often limited in out-of-hospital settings. This limits timely clinical actions and data collection for evaluating outcomes.

Furthermore, unlike obstetric teams in hospital settings, EMS personnel typically lack the equipment and training to perform gynaecological assessments such as per vaginam examination or speculum inspection. These skills are essential for identifying common sources of postpartum haemorrhages—such as retained placental tissue or birth canal lacerations—and their absence may delay accurate diagnosis and intervention in the pre-hospital setting.

To sum up, EMS personnel may lack experience, confidence, and time in diagnosing and managing early signs of PPH. Finally, incomplete documentation and a lack of real-time monitoring limit both response accuracy and data collection for evaluating outcomes.

4.6. Advances in PPH Prevention and Treatment Research

Efforts are ongoing worldwide to develop a method that is 100% effective, safe for patients, and easily accessible [33]. Such a solution would be applicable in hospital settings, suitable for home births, and used by emergency medical teams, ensuring broader reach and adaptability in diverse childbirth scenarios.

In low-resource settings, the effective use of oxytocin is often hindered by challenges related to manufacturing quality and degradation caused by inadequate cold chain management [34]. Heat-stable carbetocin (HSC) has emerged as a promising alternative, with multiple studies confirming its effectiveness in preventing postpartum haemorrhage. A single 100 mcg dose of HSC has been shown to have similar efficacy to 10 units of oxytocin [35].

While its effectiveness has also been demonstrated in caesarean deliveries, many experts remain cautiously optimistic. This is primarily due to concerns regarding the cost-effectiveness of HSC, particularly when considering its implementation in resource-constrained healthcare systems [36].

The development of a thermostable, easy-to-administer microneedle (MN) patch for oxytocin delivery holds significant potential for use by emergency medical teams, particularly in low-resource settings. This innovation addresses the logistical challenges of transporting and storing oxytocin, which requires refrigeration.

It is designed to administer 10 IU (16.8 μg) of oxytocin, providing an efficient and reliable prevention and treatment method for postpartum haemorrhage.

In emergencies, such as during home births or remote medical interventions, MN patches could provide a quick, reliable method for administering oxytocin, even by healthcare workers with limited training, such as traditional birth attendants or paramedics [37].

There is growing hope for the future in combination therapy. Numerous studies have shown that using two or more drugs in tandem increases the effectiveness of preventing postpartum haemorrhage. For example, combinations such as ergometrine plus oxytocin, carbetocin, and misoprostol plus oxytocin have proven more effective uterotonic strategies than the current standard, oxytocin alone. However, combinations like ergometrine plus oxytocin and misoprostol plus oxytocin are associated with significant side effects. As a result, there is potential for developing combined formulations that incorporate several drugs, aiming to maximize efficacy while minimizing adverse effects [38].

An emerging and effective therapy for postpartum haemorrhage involves the use of oxytocin in nasal or inhalable forms. This non-invasive delivery method has shown promise, particularly in emergency settings where rapid intervention is critical. Nasal spray formulations of uterotonics, currently under development, offer a quick and accessible alternative to traditional methods of administration, such as injections or intravenous access. These nasal sprays are especially advantageous for healthcare workers with limited training, including traditional birth attendants and emergency medical teams, who may be required to act quickly in challenging environments. By eliminating the need for needles, these spray formulations make it easier for non-specialist personnel to administer lifesaving drugs, particularly in remote or resource-limited settings. This approach holds great potential for improving the management of PPH in emergencies where time and access to medical facilities are limited [39–41].

4.7. Implications for Practice

Despite limited proof of efficacy in current studies, the routine inclusion of oxytocin in prehospital obstetric care may still be justified due to its established safety profile and strong endorsement by global authorities. The significant barriers are systemic rather than clinical. Broader inclusion of oxytocin in EMS protocols, expanded scope-of-practice for paramedics, and targeted education may improve consistency and potential outcomes. Furthermore, the promising development of heat-stable, easy-to-administer formulations (e.g., microneedle patches and nasal sprays) could significantly improve feasibility in low-resource and field settings.

4.8. Limitations

Only articles published in English were considered in the analysis. The analysed articles presented cases of the use of uterotonic drugs by emergency medical teams in prehospital care. Therefore, given the limited number of studies that met the inclusion criteria, we opted not to perform a meta-analysis, which would have quantitatively combined data from multiple studies. Instead, our findings and recommendations are based on an assessment of study quality and a synthesis of the available evidence rather than aggregated quantitative measures. The nature of these analyses limited the possibility of drawing far-reaching conclusions. The review included only four studies, all observational and geographically restricted, limiting generalizability. No randomized controlled trials were identified, and heterogeneity in research protocols and outcome reporting indicates difficulty in comparison. Additionally, variability in EMS systems and protocols across regions results in challenges in standardizing conclusions, further limiting the applicability of the findings to diverse healthcare contexts.

4.9. Future Research

Future studies should focus on evaluating standardized oxytocin administration protocols within EMS systems, ideally through prospective or controlled designs. Research should explore more up-to-date delivery systems suited to the settings context, such as non-injectable formulations. Crucially, EMS-focused guidelines for obstetric emergencies—including medication protocols—must be developed to align more closely with hospital-based standards.

5. Conclusions

While oxytocin is widely recognized as a first-line agent for preventing postpartum haemorrhage in hospital settings, its use in prehospital obstetric care remains inconsistent and under-researched. The evidence suggests no apparent reduction in PPH rates and no safety concerns when administered by EMS teams. To improve care for out-of-hospital deliveries, EMS systems should consider updating protocols to include oxytocin, invest in practical training, and advocate for the legal authority of paramedics to administer uterotonics autonomously. Future research and innovation—including novel delivery systems—are needed to close the gap between international recommendations and real-world EMS practice.

To improve care for out-of-hospital deliveries, EMS systems should include oxytocin in their protocols and align with unified international recommendations such as those from the WHO and FIGO. Applying these standardized, evidence-based protocols across prehospital systems would result in equity, enhance safety, and support frontline providers in delivering optimal care while managing obstetric emergencies. Practical training, regulatory reform, and investment in accessible uterotonic delivery options must accompany these efforts to bridge the gap between guidelines and real-world EMS practice.

Author Contributions: Conceptualisation, H.W. and M.S.; methodology, H.W., M.S. and J.S.; investigation, H.W., M.S. and J.S.; data curation, H.W., M.S. and J.S.; formal analysis, H.W., M.S. and J.S.; writing—original draft preparation, H.W. and M.S.; writing—review and editing, H.W. and J.S.; supervision, J.S.; project administration, H.W. and J.S.; funding acquisition, J.S. All authors have read and agreed to the published version of the manuscript.

Funding: This research was funded by Wroclaw Medical University, Wroclaw, Poland (grant SUBZ.L030.25.052).

Institutional Review Board Statement: Not applicable.

Informed Consent Statement: Not applicable.

Data Availability Statement: All data on which the review is based are available in public databases with references provided in the section. Detailed methodology for literature selection is described in Section 2.

Conflicts of Interest: The authors declare no conflicts of interest.

References

1. Kassebaum, N.J.; Barber, R.M.; Bhutta, Z.A.; Dandona, L.; Gething, P.W.; Hay, S.I.; Kinfu, Y.; Larson, H.J.; Liang, X.; Lim, S.S.; et al. Global, regional, and national levels of maternal mortality, 1990–2015: A systematic analysis for the Global Burden of Disease Study 2015. *Lancet* **2016**, *388*, 1775–1812. [CrossRef]
2. WHO Recommendation on Tranexamic Acid for the Treatment of Postpartum Haemorrhage—Highlights and Key Messages. Available online: https://www.who.int/publications/i/item/WHO-RHR-17.21 (accessed on 26 November 2024).
3. ACOG. ACOG Expands Recommendations to Treat Postpartum Hemorrhage. Available online: https://www.acog.org/news/news-releases/2017/09/acog-expands-recommendations-to-treat-postpartum-hemorrhage (accessed on 26 November 2024).
4. Robinson, D.; Basso, M.; Chan, C.; Duckitt, K.; Lett, R. Corrigendum to 'Guideline No. 431: Postpartum Hemorrhage and Hemorrhagic Shock' [Journal of Obstetrics and Gynaecology Canada 2022; 44(12): 1293-1310.E1]. *J. Obstet. Gynaecol. Can.* **2024**, *46*, 102174. [CrossRef] [PubMed]
5. Begley, C.M.; Gyte, G.M.; Devane, D.; McGuire, W.; Weeks, A.; Biesty, L.M. Active versus expectant management for women in the third stage of labour. *Cochrane Database Syst. Rev.* **2019**, *2019*, CD007412. [CrossRef]
6. De Silva, M.; Mizzi, G.; Potts, E.; Webb, J.; Thyer, E.; Naidoo, N. Tranexamic acid versus oxytocin for primary postpartum Haemorrhage in the out-of-hospital setting: A systematic review with implications for rural practice. *Aust. J. Rural. Health* **2024**, *32*, 227–235. [CrossRef]
7. Wiciak, H.; Strózik, M.; Smereka, A.; Fuchs, T.; Smereka, J. Situations in Which Oxytocin Was Administrated by Paramedics in Out-of-Hospital Births: A Retrospective Analysis over Six Years in the Polish Population. *J. Clin. Med.* **2024**, *13*, 7175. [CrossRef]
8. Schultz, B.V.; Hall, S.; Parker, L.; Rashford, S.; Bosley, E. Epidemiology of Oxytocin Administration in Out-of-Hospital Births Attended by Paramedics. *Prehospital Emerg. Care* **2020**, *25*, 412–417. [CrossRef] [PubMed]
9. Klemettilä, E.; Rahkonen, L.; Nuutila, M.; Lääperi, M.; Harve-Rytsälä, H. Role of oxytocin in prevention of postpartum hemorrhage in unplanned out-of-hospital deliveries treated by emergency medical services. *Acta Obstet. Gynecol. Scand.* **2020**, *99*, 901–908. [CrossRef] [PubMed]

10. Beaird, D.T.; Ladd, M.; Jenkins, S.M.; Kahwaji, C.I. *EMS Prehospital Deliveries*; StatPearls: Treasure Island, FL, USA, 2023. Available online: https://www.ncbi.nlm.nih.gov/books/NBK525996/ (accessed on 11 November 2024).
11. Flanagan, B.; Lord, B.; Barnes, M. Is unplanned out-of-hospital birth managed by paramedics infrequent, normal and uncomplicated? *BMC Pregnancy Childbirth* **2017**, *17*, 436. [CrossRef]
12. Khazaei, A.; Esmaeili, M.; Navab, E. The Most and Least Stressful Prehospital Emergencies from Emergency Medical Technicians' View Point; a Cross-Sectional Study. *Arch. Acad. Emerg. Med.* **2019**, *7*, e20. [CrossRef]
13. Galková, G.; Böhm, P.; Hon, Z.; Heřman, T.; Doubrava, R.; Navrátil, L. Comparison of Frequency of Home Births in the Member States of the EU Between 2015 and 2019. *Glob. Pediatr. Health* **2022**, *9*, 2333794X211070916. [CrossRef]
14. McLelland, G.; McKenna, L.; Morgans, A.; Smith, K. Epidemiology of unplanned out-of-hospital births attended by paramedics. *BMC Pregnancy Childbirth* **2018**, *18*, 15. [CrossRef]
15. Heys, S.; Main, C.; Humphreys, A.; Torrance, R. Displaced risk. Keeping mothers and babies safe: A UK ambulance service lens. *Br. Paramedic J.* **2023**, *8*, 52–56. [CrossRef]
16. Strózik, M.; Wiciak, H.; Raczyński, A.; Smereka, J. Emergency medical team interventions in Poland during out-of-hospital deliveries: A retrospective analysis. *Adv. Clin. Exp. Med.* **2024**. *Online ahead of print*. [CrossRef] [PubMed]
17. Vagle, H.; Haukeland, G.T.; Dahl, B.; Aasheim, V.; Vik, E.S. Emergency medical technicians' experiences with unplanned births outside institutions: A qualitative interview study. *Nurs. Open* **2019**, *6*, 1542–1550. [CrossRef]
18. Greenaway, M. Prophylactic uterotonics in the prevention of primary postpartum haemorrhage for unplanned out-of-hospital births: A literature review. *Br. Paramed. J.* **2019**, *3*, 15–22. [CrossRef] [PubMed]
19. Ovaskainen, K.; Ojala, R.; Tihtonen, K.; Gissler, M.; Luukkaala, T.; Tammela, O. Unplanned out-of-hospital deliveries in Finland: A national register study on incidence, characteristics and maternal and infant outcomes. *Acta Obstet. Gynecol. Scand.* **2020**, *99*, 1691–1699. [CrossRef] [PubMed]
20. Jenneker, M.; Maharaj, N.R. Perinatal Outcomes in Babies Born before Arrival at Prince Mshiyeni Memorial Hospital in Durban, South Africa. *Obstet. Gynecol. Int.* **2022**, *2022*, 2316490. [CrossRef]
21. Goodwin, L.; Kirby, K.; McClelland, G.; Beach, E.; Bedson, A.; Benger, J.R.; Deave, T.; Osborne, R.; McAdam, H.; McKeon-Carter, R.; et al. Inequalities in birth before arrival at hospital in South West England: A multimethods study of neonatal hypothermia and emergency medical services call-handler advice. *BMJ Open* **2024**, *14*, e081106-11. [CrossRef]
22. Gunnarsson, B.; Fasting, S.; Skogvoll, E.; Smárason, A.K.; Salvesen, K.Å. Why babies die in unplanned out-of-institution births: An enquiry into perinatal deaths in Norway 1999–2013. *Acta Obstet. Gynecol. Scand.* **2017**, *96*, 326–333. [CrossRef]
23. Yeshaneh, A.; Tadele, B.; Dessalew, B.; Alemayehu, M.; Wolde, A.; Adane, A.; Shitu, S.; Abebe, H.; Adane, D. Incidence and predictors of mortality among neonates referred to comprehensive and specialized hospitals in Amhara regional state, North Ethiopia: A prospective follow-up study. *Ital. J. Pediatr.* **2021**, *47*, 186. [CrossRef]
24. Ognean, M.L.; Coțovanu, B.; Teacoe, D.A.; Radu, I.A.; Todor, S.B.; Ichim, C.; Mureșan, I.C.; Boicean, A.-G.; Galiș, R.; Cucerea, M. Identification of the Best Predictive Model for Mortality in Outborn Neonates—Retrospective Cohort Study. *Healthcare* **2023**, *11*, 3131. [CrossRef]
25. Singh, S.; Agrawal, R.; Das, A.; Sahu, R.; Agrawal, G. Predictors of Neonatal Mortality: A Retrospective Cross-Sectional Study from the Special Newborn Care Unit of a Tertiary Care Hospital. *Cureus* **2023**, *15*, e37143. [CrossRef]
26. McLelland, G.; McKenna, L.; Morgans, A.; Smith, K. Paramedics' involvement in planned home birth: A one-year case study. *Midwifery* **2016**, *38*, 71–77. [CrossRef] [PubMed]
27. Leduc, D.; Senikas, V.; Lalonde, A.B.; Ballerman, C.; Biringer, A.; Delaney, M.; Duperron, L.; Girard, I.; Jones, D.; Lee, L.S.-Y.; et al. Active Management of the Third Stage of Labour: Prevention and Treatment of Postpartum Hemorrhage. *J. Obstet. Gynaecol. Can.* **2009**, *31*, 980–993. [CrossRef] [PubMed]
28. WHO's Department of Reproductive Health and Research. *WHO Recommendations for the Prevention and Treatment of Postpartum Haemorrhage*; World Health Organization: Rome, Italy, 2012; p. 41. Available online: https://www.who.int/publications/i/item/9789241548502 (accessed on 11 November 2024).
29. Ranzcog, Management of Postpartum Haemorrhage (PPH). November 2021. Available online: https://ranzcog.edu.au/wp-content/uploads/Management-Postpartum-Haemorrhage.pdf (accessed on 11 November 2024).
30. Escobar, M.F.; Nassar, A.H.; Theron, G.; Barnea, E.R.; Nicholson, W.; Ramasauskaite, D.; Lloyd, I.; Chandraharan, E.; Miller, S.; Burke, T.; et al. FIGO recommendations on the management of postpartum hemorrhage *Int. J. Gynecol. Obstet.* **2022**, *157* (Suppl. 1), 3–50. [CrossRef]
31. Postpartum Hemorrhage. Committee on Practice Bulletins-Obstetrics Practice Bulletin No. 183. *Obstet. Gynecol.* **2017**, *130*, e168–e186. [CrossRef]
32. Kietaibl, S.; Ahmed, A.; Afshari, A.; Albaladejo, P.; Aldecoa, C.; Barauskas, G.; De Robertis, E.; Faraoni, D.; Filipescu, D.C.; Fries, D.; et al. Management of severe peri-operative bleeding: Guidelines from the European Society of Anaesthesiology and Intensive Care. *Eur. J. Anaesthesiol.* **2023**, *40*, 226–304. [CrossRef]

33. Hofmeyr, G.J. Novel concepts and improvisation for treating postpartum haemorrhage: A narrative review of emerging techniques. *Reprod. Health* **2023**, *20*, 116. [CrossRef]
34. Gallos, I.D.; Coomarasamy, A. Carbetocin: Worth the extra expense? *Best Pract. Res. Clin. Obstet. Gynaecol.* **2019**, *61*, 55–65. [CrossRef]
35. Widmer, M.; Piaggio, G.; Nguyen, T.M.; Osoti, A.; Owa, O.O.; Misra, S.; Coomarasamy, A.; Abdel-Aleem, H.; Mallapur, A.A.; Qureshi, Z.; et al. Heat-Stable Carbetocin versus Oxytocin to Prevent Hemorrhage after Vaginal Birth. *N. Engl. J. Med.* **2018**, *379*, 743–752. [CrossRef]
36. Voon, H.Y.; Suharjono, H.N.; Shafie, A.A.; Bujang, M.A. Carbetocin versus oxytocin for the prevention of postpartum hemorrhage: A meta-analysis of randomized controlled trials in cesarean deliveries. *Taiwan. J. Obstet. Gynecol.* **2018**, *57*, 332–339. [CrossRef] [PubMed]
37. Gomaa, Y.; Kolluru, C.; Milewski, M.; Lee, D.; Zhang, J.; Saklatvala, R.; Prausnitz, M.R. Development of a thermostable oxytocin microneedle patch. *J. Control. Release* **2021**, *337*, 81–89. [CrossRef]
38. Gallos, I.; Williams, H.; Price, M.; Pickering, K.; Merriel, A.; Tobias, A.; Lissauer, D.; Gee, H.; Tunçalp, Ö.; Gyte, G.; et al. Uterotonic drugs to prevent postpartum haemorrhage: A network meta-analysis. *Health Technol. Assess.* **2019**, *23*, 1–356. [CrossRef] [PubMed]
39. McDougall, A.R.; Goldstein, M.; Tuttle, A.; Ammerdorffer, A.; Rushwan, S.; Hastie, R.; Gülmezoglu, A.M.; Vogel, J.P. Innovations in the prevention and treatment of postpartum hemorrhage: Analysis of a novel medicines development pipeline database. *Int. J. Gynecol. Obstet.* **2022**, *158*, 31–39. [CrossRef] [PubMed]
40. Carvalho, N.; Hoque, M.E.; Oliver, V.L.; Byrne, A.; Kermode, M.; Lambert, P.; McIntosh, M.P.; Morgan, A. Cost-effectiveness of inhaled oxytocin for prevention of postpartum haemorrhage: A modelling study applied to two high burden settings. *BMC Med.* **2020**, *18*, 1–18. [CrossRef]
41. Gajewska-Knapik, K.; Kumar, S.; Sutton-Cole, A.; Palmer, K.R.; Cahn, A.; Gibson, R.A.; Kirkpatrick, C.; Parry, S.; Schneider, I.; Siederer, S.; et al. Pharmacokinetics and safety of inhaled oxytocin compared with intramuscular oxytocin in women in the third stage of labour: A randomized open-label study. *Br. J. Clin. Pharmacol.* **2023**, *89*, 3681–3689. [CrossRef]

healthcare

MDPI

Case Report

The Role of Paramedics in Diagnosing Sandifer's Syndrome

Michał Wójcik [1,*], Damian Krysiak [1], Piotr Babik [1], Łukasz Suchanek [1], Michał Ćwiertnia [1,2], Joanna Trojak-Piętka [1], Marek Kawecki [1], Wioletta Pollok-Waksmańska [3], Monika Mikulska [1] and Tomasz Ilczak [1,2]

[1] Department of Emergency Medicine, Faculty of Health Sciences, University of Bielsko-Biala, 43-309 Bielsko-Biała, Poland; dkrysiak@ubb.edu.pl (D.K.); pbabik@ubb.edu.pl (P.B.); lsuchanek@ubb.edu.pl (Ł.S.); mcwiertnia@ubb.edu.pl (M.Ć.); jpietka@ubb.edu.pl (J.T.-P.); mkawecki@ubb.edu.pl (M.K.); mmikulska@ubb.edu.pl (M.M.); tilczak@ubb.edu.pl (T.I.)

[2] European Pre-Hospital Research Network, Nottingham NG11 8NS, UK

[3] Department of Public Health, Faculty of Health Sciences, University of Bielsko-Biala, 43-309 Bielsko-Biała, Poland; wwaksmanska@ubb.edu.pl

* Correspondence: miwojcik@ubb.edu.pl; Tel.: +48-338279199

Abstract: Background: Sandifer's syndrome is an uncharacteristic symptom of gastroesophageal reflux disease (GERD). It is often misdiagnosed as epilepsy. Paramedics can play a crucial role in recognising the differences between Sandifer's syndrome and epilepsy. Therefore, education is important to reduce the likelihood of misdiagnosis and the mistreatment of patients. This purpose of this study is to provides information and guidelines for collecting patients' medical history and identifying the most common symptoms, which support pre-hospital suspicion of Sandifer's syndrome. **Methods:** The study consisted of a clinical case study, concerning the management of the emergency team, in a 7-week-old child with symptoms indicative of an epileptic seizure. **Results:** The clinical case analysis showed that a thorough examination of the patient helped to rule out epilepsy in the child and observed the characteristic symptoms of Sandifer syndrome. While assisting the child, a rare symptom of apnoea was also observed. **Conclusions**: The role of the paramedics in diagnosing Sandifer's syndrome can be crucial. Their experience and knowledge of emergency situations, as well as correctly conducted tests during and immediately after ailment symptoms, can provide medical teams with key information that can help in making a correct diagnosis. The presented framework can be helpful. In the majority of cases, a correct diagnosis leads to the complete cessation of symptoms and lowers the risk of side effects from unnecessarily applied anti-epilepsy medication.

Keywords: Sandifer's syndrome; paediatric; seizures; gastroesophageal reflux; emergency medical service; vagus nerve

1. Introduction

According to statistics from the Polish Central Statistical Office, emergency response teams (ERTs) intervened almost 3.1 million times in 2022 [1]. Interventions involving children and adolescents below 18 years of age constituted only 6.7% of this figure, which corresponds to European estimates, accounting for 6–10% of all emergency department patients [2]. Research conducted in simulated conditions on a group of paramedics working in Switzerland confirmed that interventions which involve providing assistance to children are highly stressful for medical personnel. This may be related to time pressure, limited experience with paediatric patients, and, in particular, the need to calculate and properly administer specific drug doses [3]. It is estimated that chronic diseases in paediatric patients affect 30% of children around the world [4]. According to various sources, gastroesophageal reflux affects, depending on age, around 10% of children, and among infants, this percentage rises even to 80 to 90%. Sandifer's syndrome, which is a non-specific set of symptoms, affects only 1% of these children [5]. Due to the atypical symptoms suggesting a problem of neurological and not gastrological origin, it may be the reason for requesting an ERT intervention and can be connected to unnecessary pharmacotherapy, erroneous procedures, and extended diagnosis. A thorough examination and the collection of a detailed medical history can help members of an emergency medical team to make the correct diagnosis and implement the right management [5].

The aim of this article is to present a rare disease entity occurring among children, which is Sandifer's syndrome. The article presents the difficulties that emergency medical teams may encounter when providing assistance to a patient with this disease.

2. Gastroesophageal Reflux and Gastroesophageal Reflux Disease

Gastroesophageal reflux (GER) is a very common phenomenon, affecting, depending on the source, from about half to even two-thirds of all infants [6,7]. The backflow of stomach contents into the oesophagus is a physiological process that occurs several times a day in healthy infants, children, and adults [7]. The causes vary with age. In older children and adults, dysfunction in the lower oesophageal sphincter is the primary factor, while in infancy, the pressure difference between the stomach and oesophagus also plays a significant role [8]. In 2009, the North American Society for Pediatric Gastroenterology, Hepatology, and Nutrition (NASPGHAN) and the European Society for Paediatric Gastroenterology, Hepatology, and Nutrition (ESPGHAN) issued a joint statement distinguishing gastroesophageal reflux disease (GERD) from GER (despite these terms often being used interchangeably). GERD is defined as the occurrence of troublesome symptoms and complications resulting from GER [7,9]. In children, particularly those who have not yet developed verbal communication skills, it is often impossible to determine whether "troublesome symptoms" are present. Therefore, different symptoms of GERD are assigned depending on the patient's age. The most common symptoms in infants include recurrent vomiting, feeding aversion, frequent choking, as well as irritability and frequent crying. In adults and older children, the primary symptoms include recurrent vomiting, abdominal or chest pain with a burning sensation, primarily heartburn, and swallowing disorders (dysphagia) [7,9]. Since 2009, the definition has not been updated. Based on this definition, guidelines were developed, initially by the National Institute for Health and Care Excellence (NICE) in 2015, and later updated in 2018 with joint recommendations by the NASPGHAN and ESPGHAN [9,10].

3. What Is Sandifer's Syndrome and What Are the Symptoms?

The illness currently known as Sandifer's syndrome was first described in the 1960s by the Austrian neurologist Marcel Kinsbourn. It takes its name from a British doctor, Paul Sandifer, who was the first to notice a correlation between the occurrence of torticollis in children after a meal [11,12]. According to the definition, it is a non-specific, extraoesophageal manifestation of gastroesophageal reflux disease (GERD), accompanied by neurological symptoms similar to epileptic seizures [12]. In the literature, it is most commonly described as dystonia, the occurrence of involuntary movements located around the head, neck, and torso, as well as shaking, problems with breathing, eye rotation and a decrease in muscle tone [11,13]. In contrast to epileptic seizures, during seizures in Sandifer's syndrome, there is no rhythmic or clonic component, and the symptoms do not affect the limbs [5,11,12]. In addition, symptomatic episodes do not occur during sleep, and patients are conscious and partially react to stimuli [5]. The next important piece of information that makes it possible to distinguish the syndrome is the time when seizures occur: usually a short time after feeding [14]. In addition to the symptoms ascribed to Sandifer's syndrome, depending on age, children will have various gastroesophageal reflux disease (GERD) symptoms. In infants, these include crying and irritation, unwillingness to feed, and further consequences involving problems with gaining weight and recurrent respiratory tract infections, including lung infections [15]. In older children, the symptoms are identical to those that occur in adults, that is, burping, heartburn, vomiting, a chronic cough, chronic stridor and wheezing, recurrent lung infections, and apnoea [5,15].

4. Aetiology

Despite being recognised for many years, the exact cause of these symptoms remains unknown. Some authors suggest that dystonia and the body position are adopted by children unconsciously and that it is a learned behaviour that aims to ease discomfort at the moment of gastric reflux [5]. It has been proven that the adopted position accelerates the process of emptying the stomach [16]. However, this explains the occurrence of only some of the symptoms. The latest hypothesis is based on the position that it is a response of the vagus nerve, with its nerve endings being irritated by the released acidic content [16]. The vagus nerve is the longest cranial nerve and controls the most important functions of the human body. These include heart rate, blood pressure, breathing, and intestinal motility, as well as swallowing, the cough reflex, and the immunological response as a reaction to disease [17]. It is also responsible for the functioning of some muscles [17]. The vagus nerve's fibres consist of both sensory neurons (around 80%) and motor and parasympathetic neurons. It is responsible for innervation of the throat, larynx, and heart, parts of the respiratory tract including the lungs, and parts of the digestive tract: the oesophagus, stomach, liver, pancreas, small intestine, and proximal colon [18,19]. There is ongoing research and debate as to whether this does not also include the spleen, kidneys, adrenal glands, and reproductive organs. It continues to be the subject of many discussions. The complex structure of the vagus nerve allows for the implementation of therapies in patients, acting on it to treat various medical conditions [19]. The most common example is the stimulation of this nerve during supraventricular tachycardia, which is used to slow the heart rate. Increasingly, targeted electrical impulses are being used to treat a variety of clinical disorders, such as heart failure, migraine, and inflammatory bowel disease [17]. Given the complexity of the vagus nerve and the nonspecific, often seemingly unrelated symptoms of Sandifer's syndrome, it seems justified to search for the cause in its irritation.

5. Diagnostics and Treatment

In medical ERT practice, it is not possible to make a clear diagnosis due to limited diagnostic capabilities. However, due to the fact that an ERT is called for at the moment when symptoms appear, paramedics are able to notice the difference between symptoms of Sandifer's syndrome and those of typical epileptic seizures, which is not possible in the case of planned visits to specialist clinics. An additional difficulty in making a correct diagnosis is that the child's parents often do not have specialist medical knowledge, and they are also subjected to the additional factor of stress when the symptoms appear. Then, interviewing them is incomplete, chaotic and not very accurate. An additional difficulty is the impossibility of interviewing the child directly. This often directs diagnosis and treatment towards epileptic seizures [13]. This involves costly tests of the nervous system in which deviations from the norm are not found, extending the time taken to give the correct diagnosis and apply appropriate treatment, and above all, the use of antiepileptic medicines that do not have a neutral effect on the body may occur. In research conducted by Kotagala et al. [20] from the university of Cleveland in 1989–1995, among a group of

883 children on an epilepsy monitoring ward, 134 children were found not to have epilepsy. In the youngest age group (2–5 years), Sandifer's syndrome was one of the three mostly frequently diagnosed diseases. Therefore, differential diagnosis performed in a hospital or in a specialist clinic is very important. In the initial diagnostic stage, medical interviews play a crucial role. Various questionnaires have been created to assess the frequency and intensity of symptoms, such as the Gastroesophageal Reflux Disease Health-Related Quality of Life (GERD-HRQL) Questionnaire or the Gastrointestinal Symptom Rating Scale (GSRS) [21]. These are effective methods for conducting subjective assessments but may be ineffective in the youngest patients. Nonetheless, it is believed that a well-conducted medical interview is sufficient to confirm GERD, and additional tests such as contrast radiography of the upper gastrointestinal tract, esophageal pH monitoring, gastroesophageal scintigraphy, or esophageal endoscopy with biopsy are not necessary. However, there may be additional concerning symptoms that require extended diagnostics. These include gastrointestinal bleeding, hepatosplenomegaly, persistent and severe vomiting, fever, abnormal head size, and bulging fontanelle [7]. Differentiating Sandifer's syndrome from epileptic seizures is primarily based on EEG recordings and neuroimaging diagnostics of the central nervous system. Once a diagnosis has been made, the cure is based on treatment of GERD, after which the symptoms of Sandifer's syndrome disappear. Treatment does not only consist of pharmacotherapy; initially, a modification to the diet is applied as well as education for the parents regarding feeding habits. An example of this is not giving the child excessively large meals and preventing the child from adopting a reclining position immediately after food [5]. Only when non-pharmacological methods do not bring results should pharmacological treatment be applied. The principal method is to use proton pump inhibitors and H2 blockers, after which, in most cases, the symptoms disappear [5,13]. Only in a few cases is surgical intervention or enteral feeding necessary [13]. To date, no recommendations and guidelines have been developed anywhere in the world for emergency response teams. In practice, when a patient has confirmed Sandifer's syndrome, a crucial part of the procedure is the appropriate examination of the child to exclude other emergency conditions, including, above all, epileptic seizures, as well as ceasing the administration of benzodiazepine and the possible implementation of treatment for accompanying symptoms. If breathing problems occur, it may be necessary to assist with breathing. The patient should always be transported to hospital. This will enable broader diagnosis and possible modification to the treatment implemented so far [13].

6. Case Study Description

The parents of an unconscious seven-week-old boy, weighing approximately 5500 g, returned to the emergency medical service (EMS) station. The reason for their visit was their unsuccessful attempts to wake the boy, which lasted about 10 min. Due to the short distance from their home to the EMS station, the parents decided to seek help on their own. One member the EMS team immediately assessed the patient's condition following the ABCDE protocol recommended by the European Resuscitation Council guidelines, while the other went to obtain the equipment needed to conduct paediatric advanced life support. The assessment of airway patency revealed no obstruction or risk of obstruction. In response to a painful stimulus, the boy displayed a facial grimace. He also briefly opened his eyes. His respiratory rate was approximately 30 breaths per minute, with no signs of respiratory distress, accessory muscle use, nasal flaring, or abnormal breath sounds. Auscultation revealed symmetrical physiological vesicular breath sounds over the lung fields. His heart rate was regular, with distinct heart sounds and a palpable brachial pulse at approximately 140 beats per minute. His blood pressure was within the normal range for his age. The examination showed that the child's skin was pink, adequately moist, and of a normal temperature, with a capillary refill time of less than 2 s. The tympanic membrane temperature measured 36.8 °C. During the patient examinations, a medical history was obtained from the child's parents. From the conversation, it was found that the child had been discharged from the neurology department of a children's hospital a few days earlier after previously staying in intensive care due to suspected epilepsy. The mother had the hospital discharge summary and handed it to the paramedics. During hospitalisation, imaging studies (MRI, ultrasound), laboratory tests, and functional tests (EEG) were performed, all of which showed no pathological disorder, effectively ruling out epilepsy The attending neurologist, based on the conducted diagnostics, referred the child to a neurology and gastroenterology clinic upon discharge. The referral to the gastroenterology clinic was mainly due to the doctor's suspicion of Sandifer's syndrome. The parents, following recommendations, contacted a gastroenterology clinic and were awaiting their scheduled appointment. Neither the child nor the mother were on any long-term medications, and the child had been breastfed a maximum of two hours before falling asleep. During the medical history assessment, the paramedics observed a sudden change in the child's body position, involving the head, neck, and torso. The child's body was arched in a posture resembling an inverted "U". The paramedics noted no increased muscle tone in the limbs. Moments later, they observed that the child's chest stopped rising. The child's breathing was reassessed and found to have ceased. One of the EMS team members, acting as the team leader, instructed the second paramedic to prepare a self-inflating bag. While preparing the equipment, the child was listened to again and no vesicular murmur was found, accompanied by a continued regular heartbeat and no drop in oxygen saturation. The child's skin remained pink, warm, and properly hydrated. A painful stimulus was applied to stimulate breathing, but without effect. After approximately 30 s, spontaneous respiration resumed at a rate of 30 to 35 breaths per minute, eliminating the need for assisted ventilation. The unnatural body posture disappeared along with the apnea, and the child began spontaneously opening his eyes. A neurological examination showed no abnormalities: muscle strength was symmetrically preserved, the child responded to pain stimuli with crying, no cranial nerve dysfunction was observed, and no signs of meningeal irritation or fever were present. From that moment on, the child's condition remained unchanged. Based on the observed symptoms, collected medical history, and previous hospital tests, the EMS team confirmed the physicians' suspicions, identifying characteristic features of Sandifer's syndrome. The child was transported to the nearest paediatric hospital. During transport, the paramedic informed the hospital staff about the child's condition and estimated time of arrival. Further observation and diagnostics conducted in the paediatric ward and gastroenterology clinic confirmed later the diagnosis of Sandifer's syndrome, validating the EMS team's initial suspicions.

7. Conclusions

The role of paramedics in diagnosing Sandifer's syndrome can be crucial. Their experience and knowledge of emergency situations, as well as correctly conducted tests during and immediately after ailment symptoms, can provide the team of doctors with key information that can help in making a correct diagnosis. To maximise the chances of making an accurate diagnosis, an acronym was created to identify the most common shared characteristics (Figure 1).

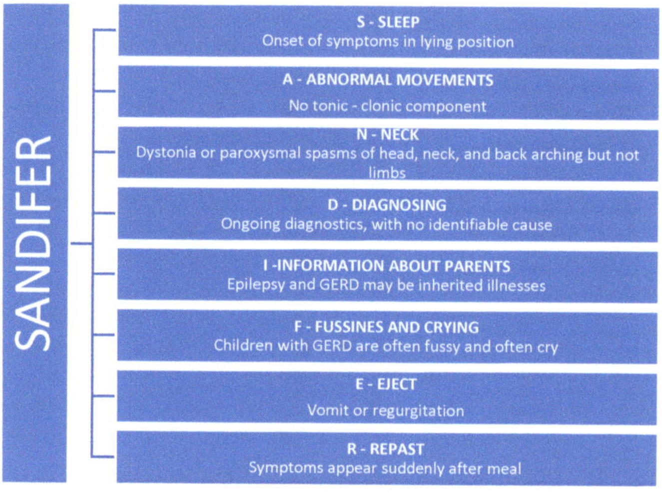

Figure 1. Scheme containing key information for considering diagnosis of Sandifer's syndrome.

This pattern for conducting a medical interview is intended to serve as a guideline for conversations with the patient's parents and should not be considered a substitute for clinical assessment or applied to all patients. The prehospital diagnosis of Sandifer's syndrome requires a detailed medical history, including information about the type of food and time since the last feeding, the position in which the patient was in when symptoms appeared, chronic illnesses of the parents, and, in the case of breastfeeding, any medications taken by the mother. Key characteristic elements to consider include frequent regurgitation, feeding aversion, and the occurrence of symptoms after meals or in a lying position. Additionally, it is crucial to differentiate Sandifer's syndrome from a typical epileptic seizure: the patient responds to stimulation (especially painful stimulation), there is no tonic–clonic component, and symptoms mainly affect the head, neck, and chest, without involving the limbs. These findings strongly suggest Sandifer's syndrome. However, confirmation of the diagnosis requires additional in-hospital examination. The clinical case described presented not only the characteristic features of Sandifer's syndrome but also the rarely described apnea, which lasted for nearly half a minute. In the majority of cases, a correct diagnosis leads to the complete cessation of symptoms and lowers the risk of side effects from unnecessarily applied anti-epilepsy medication and medical procedures, which occurred in this case. Therefore, the education of medical personnel should include topics related to the management of patients with Sandifer's syndrome.

Author Contributions: M.W.—conceptualisation, data curation, formal analysis, investigation, methodology, project administration, resources, validation, visualisation, writing—original draft, writing—review and editing, supervision; D.K.—data curation, methodology, visualisation, writing—original draft; P.B.—data curation, methodology, visualisation, writing—original draft; Ł.S.—data curation, methodology, visualisation, writing—original draft; M.Ć.—conceptualisation, writing—review and editing, supervision; J.T.-P.—data curation, project administration; M.K.—supervision; W.P.-W.—supervision; M.M.—supervision; T.I.—conceptualisation, supervision. All authors have read and agreed to the published version of the manuscript.

Funding: This research received no external funding.

Institutional Review Board Statement: Not applicable.

Informed Consent Statement: The data collected for analysis do not allow for the identification of participants in any way, nor do they violate their legal and ethical rights.

Data Availability Statement: The datasets used and/or analysed during the current study are available from the corresponding author on reasonable request.

Conflicts of Interest: The authors declare no conflicts of interest.

References

1. Polish Central Statistical Office. *Emergency Care and Medical Rescue in 2022*; Polish Central Statistical Office: Cracow, Poland, 2023.
2. Tan, C.D.; Vermont, C.L.; Zachariasse, J.M.; von Both, U.; Eleftheriou, I.; Emonts, M.; van der Flier, M.; Herberg, J.; Kohlmaier, B.; Levin, M.; et al. PERFORM consortium (Personalised Risk assessment in febrile children to optimize Real-life Management across the European Union). Emergency medical services utilisation among febrile children attending emergency departments across Europe: An observational multicentre study. *Eur. J. Paediatr.* **2023**, *182*, 3939–3947. [CrossRef]
3. Lacour, M.; Bloudeau, L.; Combescure, C.; Haddad, K.; Hugon, F.; Suppan, L.; Rodieux, F.; Lovis, C.; Gervaix, A.; Ehrler, F.; et al. PedAMINES Prehospital Group. Impact of a Mobile App on Paramedics' Perceived and Physiologic Stress Response During Simulated Prehospital Pediatric Cardiopulmonary Resuscitation: Study Nested Within a Multicenter Randomized Controlled Trial. *JMIR Mhealth Uhealth* **2021**, *9*, e31748. [CrossRef] [PubMed]
4. Pop-Jordanova, N. Chronic Diseases in Children as a Challenge for Parenting. *Pril. Makedon. Akad. Na Nauk. I Umet. Oddelenie Za Med. Nauk.* **2023**, *44*, 27–36. [CrossRef] [PubMed]
5. Patil, S.; Tas, V. Sandifer Syndrome. In *StatPearls [Internet]*; StatPearls Publishing: Treasure Island, FL, USA, 2025. [PubMed]
6. Harris, J.; Chorath, K.; Balar, E.; Xu, K.; Naik, A.; Moreira, A.; Rajasekaran, K. Clinical Practice Guidelines on Pediatric. Gastroesophageal Reflux Disease: A Systematic Quality Appraisal of International Guidelines. *Pediatr. Gastroenterol. Hepatol. Nutr.* **2022**, *25*, 109–120. [CrossRef] [PubMed]
7. Lightdale, J.R.; Gremse, D.A. Section on Gastroenterology, Hepatology, and Nutrition. Gastroesophageal reflux: Management guidance for the pediatrician. *Pediatrics* **2013**, *131*, e1684–e1695. [CrossRef] [PubMed]
8. Sawyer, C.; Sanghavi, R.; Ortigoza, E.B. Neonatal gastroesophageal reflux. *Early Hum. Dev.* **2022**, *171*, 105600. [CrossRef] [PubMed]
9. Rosen, R.; Vandenplas, Y.; Singendonk, M.; Cabana, M.; DiLorenzo, C.; Gottrand, F.; Gupta, S.; Langendam, M.; Staiano, A.; Thapar, N.; et al. Pediatric Gastroesophageal Reflux Clinical Practice Guidelines: Joint Recommendations of the North American Society for Pediatric Gastroenterology, Hepatology, and Nutrition and the European Society for Pediatric Gastroenterology, Hepatology, and Nutrition. *J. Pediatr. Gastroenterol. Nutr.* **2018**, *66*, 516–554. [CrossRef] [PubMed]
10. Davies, I.; Burman-Roy, S.; Murphy, M.S. Guideline Development Group. Gastro-oesophageal reflux disease in children: NICE guidance. *BMJ (Clin. Res. Ed.)* **2015**, *350*, g7703. [CrossRef]
11. Moore, D.M.; Rizzolo, D. Sandifer syndrome. *JAAPA Off. J. Am. Acad. Physician Assist.* **2018**, *31*, 18–22. [CrossRef] [PubMed]
12. Shrestha, A.B.; Rijal, P.; Sapkota, U.H.; Pokharel, P.; Shrestha, S. Sandifer Syndrome: A Case Report. *J. Nepal Med. Assoc.* **2021**, *59*, 1066–1068. [CrossRef] [PubMed]
13. Mindlina, I. Diagnosis and management of Sandifer syndrome in children with intractable neurological symptoms. *Eur. J. Paediatr.* **2020**, *179*, 243–250. [CrossRef] [PubMed]
14. Sharif, A.; Carr, L.; Saliakellis, E.; Chakraborty, H. Paroxysmal head drops with ataxia-like symptoms presenting as Sandifer syndrome in a 3-year old girl. *BMJ Case Rep.* **2020**, *13*, e230989. [CrossRef] [PubMed]
15. Mousa, H.; Hassan, M. Gastroesophageal Reflux Disease. *Pediatr. Clin. N. Am.* **2017**, *64*, 487–505. [CrossRef] [PubMed]
16. Iwańczak, B.; Kosmowska-Miśków, A.; Mowszet, K. Występowanie zespołu Sandifera w chorobie refluksowej przełyku u dzieci-opis trzech przypadków. *Przegląd Gastroenterol.* **2009**, *4*, 103–107.
17. Prescott, S.L.; Liberles, S.D. Internal senses of the vagus nerve. *Neuron* **2022**, *110*, 579–599. [CrossRef] [PubMed]
18. Butt, M.F.; Albusoda, A.; Farmer, A.D.; Aziz, Q. The anatomical basis for transcutaneous auricular vagus nerve stimulation. *J Anat.* **2020**, *236*, 588–611. [CrossRef] [PubMed]
19. Thompson, N.; Mastitskaya, S.; Holder, D. Avoiding off-target effects in electrical stimulation of the cervical vagus nerve: Neuroanatomical tracing techniques to study fascicular anatomy of the vagus nerve. *J. Neurosci. Methods* **2019**, *325*, 108325. [CrossRef] [PubMed]
20. Kotagal, P.; Costa, M.; Wyllie, E.; Wolgamuth, B. Paroxysmal nonepileptic events in children and adolescents. *Pediatrics* **2002**, *110*, e46. [CrossRef] [PubMed]
21. Bąk, E.; Wojtuń, S.; Gil, J.; Dyrla, P. The meaning of selected questionnaires in assessment of quality of life in patients with gastroesophageal reflux disease. *Probl. Pielęgniarstwa* **2013**, *21*, 551–559.

healthcare

MDPI

Protocol

CALL TO ECLS—Acronym for Reporting Patients for Extracorporeal Cardiopulmonary Resuscitation Procedure from Prehospital Setting to Destination Centers

Tomasz Sanak [1,2,*], Mateusz Putowski [1,2,3], Marek Dąbrowski [4], Anna Kwinta [2,5], Katarzyna Zawisza [6], Andrzej Morajda [2] and Mateusz Puślecki [7,8]

1 Faculty of Health Sciences, Jagiellonian University Medical College, 31-008 Cracow, Poland
2 Department of Anesthesiology and Intensive Care, University Hospital in Cracow, 30-688 Cracow, Poland
3 Collegium Medicum, Jan Kochanowski University, 25-317 Kielce, Poland
4 Department of Medical Education, Poznan University of Medical Sciences, 60-806 Poznan, Poland
5 Department of Anesthesiology and Intensive Care, Jagiellonian University Medical College, 31-501 Cracow, Poland
6 Epidemiology and Preventive Medicine, Jagiellonian University Medical College, 31-034 Cracow, Poland
7 Department of Medical Rescue, Poznan University of Medical Sciences, 60-608 Poznan, Poland
8 Department of Cardiac Surgery and Transplantology, Poznan University of Medical Sciences, 61-848 Poznan, Poland
* Correspondence: tomasz.sanak@uj.edu.pl

Abstract: The acronym CALL TO ECLS has been proposed as a potential tool to support decision-making in critical communication moments when qualifying a patient for the ECPR procedure. The aim of this study is to assess the accuracy of the acronym and validate its content. Validation is crucial to ensure that the acronym is theoretically correct and includes the necessary information that must be conveyed by EMS during the qualification of a patient with out-of-hospital cardiac arrest for ECMO. A survey was conducted using the LimeSurvey platform through the Survey Research System of the Jagiellonian University Medical College over a 6-month period (from December 2022 to May 2023). Usefulness, importance, clarity, and unambiguity were rated on a 4-point Likert scale, from 1 (not useful, not important, unclear, ambiguous) to 4 (useful, important, clear, unambiguous). On the 4-point scale, the Content Validity Index (I-CVI) was calculated as the percentage of subject matter experts who rated the criterion as having a level of importance/clarity/validity/uniqueness of 3 or 4. The Scale-level Content Validity Index (S-CVI) based on the average method was computed as the average of I-CVI scores (S-CVI-AVE) for all considered criteria (protocol). The number of fully completed surveys by experts was 35, and partial completion was obtained in 63 cases. All criteria were deemed significant/useful, with I-CVI coefficients ranging from 0.87 to 0.97. Similarly, the importance of all criteria was confirmed, as all I-CVI coefficients were greater than 0.78 (ranging from 0.83 to 0.97). The average I-CVI score for the ten considered criteria in terms of usefulness/significance and importance exceeded 0.9, indicating high validity of the tool/protocol/acronym. Based on the survey results and analysis of responses provided by experts, a second version was created, incorporating additional explanations. In Criterion 10, an explanation was added—"Signs of life"—during conventional cardiopulmonary resuscitation (ROSC, motor response during CPR). It has been shown that the acronym CALL TO ECLS, according to experts, is accurate and contains the necessary content, and can serve as a system to facilitate communication between the pre-hospital environment and specialized units responsible for qualifying patients for the ECPR.

Keywords: emergency medicine; pre-hospital care; communications; checklists in emergency medicine; cardiac arrest; extracorporeal cardiopulmonary resuscitation; eCPR; cardiopulmonary resuscitation

1. Introduction

The incidence of out-of-hospital cardiac arrest (OHCA) in Europe ranges from 350,000 to 700,000 events annually, which gives an average of 55 to 113 events per 100,000 residents. Unfortunately, the overall survival rate reaches only 2% to 11% and shows regional variability [1]. Positive outcomes can be achieved in cases of sudden cardiac arrest (SCA) with an initial shockable rhythm, followed by an early defibrillation and high-quality cardiopulmonary resuscitation (CPR) aimed at minimizing interruptions in chest compression and addressing potentially reversible causes of cardiac arrest. In such cases, return of spontaneous circulation (ROSC) can occur in as many as 30% to 40% of cases [2]. For patients with refractory cardiac arrest, extracorporeal cardiopulmonary resuscitation (ECPR) may be considered. European Resuscitation Council (ERC) guidelines reflect a growing body of evidence supporting extracorporeal cardiopulmonary resuscitation as a beneficial rescue therapy for selected cardiac arrest patients when conventional advanced life support (ALS) is ineffective, and specific interventions are available within a short timeframe, such as coronary angiography and percutaneous coronary intervention, pulmonary thrombectomy for massive pulmonary embolism, or rewarming in hypothermic cardiac arrest [3,4]. CPR with extracorporeal perfusion improves blood flow and oxygenation of vital organs, as well as supporting the central nervous system, preventing irreversible organ damage and cerebral ischemia during cardiac arrest. Inclusion criteria for published studies on ECPR vary, but most often include age ranges 18–65 or 18–75, cardiac arrest in the presence of witnesses, immediate bystander CPR, initial shockable rhythm, and estimated time from the start of resuscitation to ECPR initiation (low-flow time) <60 min. A shorter low-flow time consistently correlates with improved survival [5]. Appropriate application of ECPR in OHCA increases the chances of patient survival with favorable neurological outcomes [6]. The timing of team activation and cannulation performance plays an extremely important role in this context. One of the issues that can contribute to the prolongation of the time is inadequate communication between the emergency medical team and the destination center.

Effective communication within a multidisciplinary team is crucial for enhancing patient safety and the quality of work in emergency situations [7,8]. Research has shown that communication failures may come from several reasons, including difficulties among junior team members in opening up to senior specialists due to concerns about incompetence, embarrassment, verbal reprimand, lack of prior preparation or personal non-technical skills (NTSs). Poor communication is noticeable across various healthcare settings, with a significant focus on the moment of patient handover or transfer to different departments, when it is essential to share key health information in a short timeframe [9]. Such situations often occur in the Emergency Department as well [10]. To improve and systematize communication, communication strategies containing easy-to-remember acronyms are desired. These acronyms allow for the systematic inclusion of crucial patient-related information for further therapeutic processes in a short amount of time. One of these acronyms is SBAR (situation, background, assessment, and recommendation) and AT-MIST, along with the medical history acronym SAMPLE [11–13]. In the context of this article, the pivotal point is the handover of the patient from the emergency medical team to the Emergency Department or a telephone consultation with a specialist.

Efforts should be made to shorten the patient handover time while simultaneously conveying the most pertinent health information, allowing the medical staff to adequately prepare for the patient's arrival. Our devised acronym CALL TO ECLS has been proposed as a potential tool to support decision-making in critical moments to facilitate the communication process. The validation of the acronym was conducted to ensure that it includes all necessary elements according to expert opinions to quickly and effectively qualify a patient for ECPR. Our study provides the first evidence that the proposed acronym is theoretically sound and can be implemented by emergency medical teams as a communication tool. The details of the acronym are provided in Table 1.

Table 1. Detailed description of the CALL TO ECLS acronym Version 1.0.

Acronym CALL TO ECLS	
C	Cardiac Arrest to first CPR ("no-flow interval") < 5 min
A	Age, Physical Activity
L	Life-saving interventions Performed
L	Level of end-tidal CO_2 during CPR
T	Trauma signs
O	Obtained rhythm
E	Estimated time of arrival to the hospital
C	Context of the situation
L	Life-Limiting comorbidities
S	"Signs of life" during conventional CPR

2. Objective of the Study

The objective of this study is to assess the CALL TO ECLS acronym and validate its content to ensure that the acronym encompasses an appropriate number of elements and adequately covers the scope of the studied field.

3. Materials and Methodology

The survey was designed using the LimeSurvey platform through the Survey Research System of the Jagiellonian University Medical College and was conducted over a 6-month period (from December 2022 to May 2023). The questionnaire was composed of two parts: I. Metrics (7 questions) and II. Assessment of the significance/relevance of individual elements of the CALL TO ECLS acronym (4 questions). Detailed questions are presented in Table 2. Participants were allowed to skip questions. An email containing a survey link was sent to experts specializing in Extracorporeal Life Support (ECLS). Experts were intentionally recruited from corresponding authors on PubMed, among those who have area of expertise in ECLS, as well as members of the European branch of the Extracorporeal Life Support Organization (EuroELSO).

Table 2. Survey questions.

Question	I. Metrics
1.	Please specify the country in which you work.
2.	Please provide your workplace.
3.	Please provide the level of referral of the hospital in which you work.
4.	You work as (please select from the list): a specialist in anaesthesiology and intensive care physician resident of anaesthesiology and intensive care physician of another specialty (please specify)
5.	Please provide your seniority in years
6.	What is the average annual number of qualifications for ECPR performed by you
7.	Is the calling person prepared to be able to fully report the patient's condition?
	II. Assessment of the Significance/Relevance of Individual Elements of the CALL TO ECLS Report
1.	Please rate the individual indicators on a scale from 1 to 4: • 4 means = useful/important/clear/unambiguous • 3 means = rather useful/rather important/rather clear/rather unambiguous • 2 means = rather not useful/rather not important/rather not clear/rather not unambiguous • 1 means = not useful/not important/not clear/not unambiguous

Table 2. *Cont.*

Question	I. Metrics
2.	Do you suggest including any additional point in the CALL TO ECLS report?
3.	Do you suggest deleting any existing item out of the CALL TO ECLS report?
4.	What additional parameters do you propose to add to the acronym CALL TO ECLS if the patient is reported from a Hospital Emergency Department/Trauma Center/other hospital unit?

To obtain expert evaluations of the proposed criteria, a structured validity assessment form was prepared and sent to them. This form aimed to assess the usefulness and importance of each criterion in relation to the purpose of the devised acronym, as well as the clarity and unambiguity of their phrasing. Usefulness, importance, clarity, and unambiguity were rated on a 4-point Likert scale ranging from 1 (not useful, not important, unclear, and ambiguous) to 4 (useful, important, clear, and unambiguous). Experts were also asked to propose additional criteria or suggest the removal of any of the existing ones.

4. Statistical Methods

On the 4-point scale, the Content Validity Index (I-CVI) was calculated as the percentage of subject matter experts who rated the criterion as having a level of importance/clarity/validity/uniqueness of 3 or 4. The Scale-level Content Validity Index (S-CVI) based on the average method was computed as the average of I-CVI scores (S-CVI-AVE) for all considered criteria (protocol). Additionally, the percentage of criteria that all experts rated as important (3 or 4) was calculated using the Universal Agreement among Experts (S-CVI-UA). Any I-CVI value of 0.5 or less should be excluded from the tool, as this value is unacceptable. For at least nine experts, an acceptable I-CVI is at least 0.78. An S-CVI-AVE (and S-CVI-UA) of at least 0.8 indicates an accepted value, while an S-CVI-AVE (and S-CVI-UA) of at least 0.90 indicates excellent content validity of the tool. Nevertheless, S-CVI-UA is sensitive to the number of experts, and with an increase in the number of experts, it is more likely to generate a low score. It is recommended that both indicators are presented. These are common criteria used in content validity assessments [14]. These statistical methods were used to evaluate the content validity of the CALL TO ECLS acronym and its individual elements based on expert assessments and their agreement on the importance, clarity, and relevance of the proposed criteria.

5. Results

The preliminary version of the tool was sent to 287 experts. The final number of fully completed surveys was 35, and partial completion was obtained in 63 cases. The average professional experience among the surveyed experts was 15 years (median: 12 years). Specialist doctors comprised 86% of the respondents, with 67% being specialists in anesthesiology and intensive care, 17% in emergency medicine, and 16% in cardiology/cardiac surgery. The average annual number of ECPR qualifications performed by surveyed doctors was 5.7 (median: 4). The respondents primarily came from Europe (69%, n = 68), with the majority from Poland (49%, n = 48), followed by the Czech Republic (10%, n = 10), Germany (7%, n = 7), Belgium (2%, n = 2), and Sweden (1%, n = 1). Two experts were from China and one from Japan. Twenty-seven experts did not specify their workplace.

A total of 67 respondents answered Question 7, which concerned the preparedness of the person reporting the patient's condition for ECPR qualification. Among them, 43% (n = 29) indicated that the reporting person was completely unprepared for reporting the patient's condition. Detailed results are presented in Figure 1.

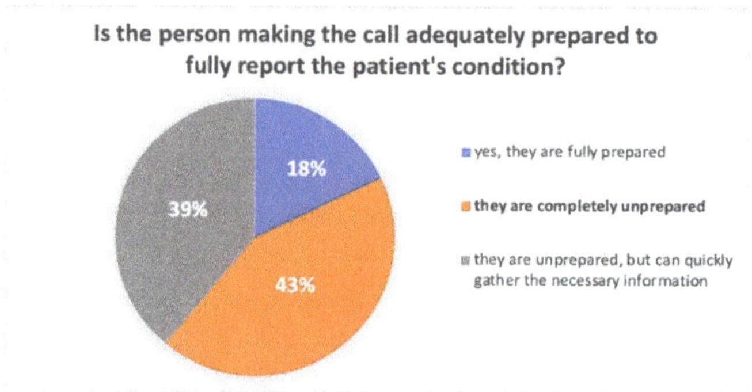

Figure 1. Is the calling person prepared to be able to fully report the patient's condition?

These findings illustrate the demographic characteristics of the surveyed experts, their experience levels, and their responses to specific questions related to the assessment of the CALL TO ECLS acronym.

All criteria were deemed significant/useful, with I-CVI coefficients ranging from 0.87 to 0.97. Similarly, the importance of all criteria was confirmed, as all I-CVI coefficients were greater than 0.78 (ranging from 0.83 to 0.97). Regarding clarity assessment, four out of ten criteria had I-CVI values slightly below 0.78. The lowest I-CVI value of 0.74 was recorded for Criterion 3, pertaining to life-saving interventions, and Criterion 10, related to "signs of life". This suggests that these criteria raised some doubts among experts regarding the clarity of the conveyed content; however, the value is far from 0.5, which would indicate the need for content reformulation. For Criteria 8 (context of the situation) and 9 (life-limiting diseases), the I-CVI values were 0.78. The lowest value for the unambiguity indicator (0.66) was observed for Criterion 10, similar to clarity assessment. Criteria 8, 9, and 2 were also rated slightly below 0.78 in terms of unambiguity (with I-CVI values of 0.71, 0.78, and 0.77, respectively).

The average I-CVI score for the ten considered criteria in terms of usefulness/significance and importance exceeded 0.9, indicating high validity of the tool/protocol/acronym. Similarly, the S-CVI-AVE values for clarity and unambiguity were higher than the required 0.80, at 0.85 and 0.81, respectively. All S-CVI-UA results were significantly below 0.8 (ranging from 0.31 for uniqueness to 0.63 for significance). Detailed results are presented in Table 3.

Table 3. Content validity of each criterion and the entire protocol in terms of usefulness/significance, importance, clarity, and unambiguity.

No.	Criterion	Usefulness		Importance		Clarity		Unambiguity	
		No. of Ratings 3 or 4	I-CVI	No. of Ratings 3 or 4	I-CVI	No. of Ratings 3 or 4	I-CVI	No. of Ratings 3 or 4	I-CVI
1	Cardiac arrest to first CPR ("no-flow interval") < 5 min	34	0.97	34	0.97	34	0.97	32	0.91
2	Age, Physical Activity	33	0.94	30	0.86	30	0.86	27	0.77
3	Life-saving interventions performed	34	0.97	33	0.94	26	0.74	29	0.83
4	Level of end-tidal CO_2 during CPR	33	0.94	31	0.89	34	0.97	33	0.94
5	Trauma signs	32	0.91	30	0.86	30	0.86	28	0.80
6	Obtained rhythm	32	0.91	32	0.91	31	0.87	32	0.91
7	Estimated time of arrival to the hospital	32	0.91	33	0.94	32	0.91	28	0.80
8	Context of the situation	31	0.87	32	0.91	27	0.77	25	0.71
9	Life-Limiting comorbidities	33	0.94	32	0.91	27	0.77	26	0.74
10	"Signs of life" during conventional CPR	32	0.91	29	0.83	26	0.74	23	0.66
	S-CVI-AVE		0.93		0.90		0.85		0.81
	S-CVI-UA		0.63		0.57		0.51		0.31

In response to Question 2 in Part II (Do you suggest including any additional point in the CALL TO ECLS report?), experts provided several significant suggestions for adding the following elements (n = 35): temperature (61%), pH value (30%), and potential poisoning (9%).

6. Modifications

Based on the survey results and analysis of responses provided by experts, a second version was created, incorporating additional explanations. In Criterion 10, an explanation was added—"Signs of life"—during conventional CPR (ROSC, motor response during CPR). Due to feedback suggesting the addition of elements to the acronym, relevant clarifications were sent. The entire algorithm refers to normothermic patients, and the lack of critical parameter analyzers in most pre-hospital medical rescue systems means that the pH parameter cannot be assessed in pre-hospital care at this time. Adding this parameter to the acronym would compromise its universality. The authors decided to include the central body temperature value; however, ongoing efforts are being made to create a dedicated acronym for reporting patients in deep hypothermia with concurrent circulatory–respiratory instability or cardiac arrest. Version 2.0 of the acronym is presented in Table 4.

Table 4. Detailed description of the CALL TO ECLS acronym Version 2.0.

	Acronym CALL TO ECLS
C	Cardiac arrest to first CPR ("no-flow interval") < 5 min
A	Age, Physical Activity
L	Life-saving interventions performed
L	Level of end-tidal CO_2 during CPR, level of central temperature
T	Trauma signs
O	Obtained rhythm
E	Estimated time of arrival to the hospital
C	Context of the situation
L	Life-Limiting comorbidities
S	"Signs of life" during conventional CPR (ROSC, motor response during CPR)

7. Discussion

An important correlation between age, initial VF/pVT rhythm, and the likelihood of survival and good neurological outcomes has been established [15–17]. Survival after ECPR is also influenced by the time between CA and the initiation of ECMO support, referred to as low-flow time, during which organ perfusion is impaired, potentially leading to multi-organ failure and cerebral ischemia [18–20]. The application of ECPR improves blood flow and oxygen delivery to tissues, preventing irreversible organ damage, especially in cases of central nervous system ischemia during CA [21]. Favorable ECPR outcomes are observed when extracorporeal techniques are applied rapidly (ideally within 1 h of CA) and when the arrest is due to potentially reversible causes. Two models of out-of-hospital ECPR implementation have been adopted worldwide [17,22]. The "Prague model" involves ECMO implantation in a hospital setting, while the "Paris model" involves ECMO implantation at the scene of the event before transporting the patient to a hospital for further intervention. The benefits of ECPR are evident when timely interventions, such as percutaneous coronary intervention in acute coronary syndrome or pulmonary thrombectomy in massive pulmonary embolism, are performed [23,24]. Correct ECPR application in refractory OHCA increases survival chances to 25–35%, with most cases achieving good neurological outcomes [25].

Extracorporeal circulation is also employed for patients after in-hospital cardiac arrest (IHCA). In these cases, factors such as time to identify CA, personnel and equipment availability significantly influence the procedure's effectiveness. IHCA patients differ significantly from OHCA patients; they are predominantly older and have multiple comorbidities. The initial shockable rhythm is less common in IHCA compared to OHCA (38% vs. 59%). Signs of deteriorating vital parameters may appear hours before CA, highlighting the importance of rapid response teams, known as Medical Emergency Teams (METs). Despite the challenges associated with IHCA patients, the use of ECPR is justified. Improved survival rates and good neurological outcomes at 3 months post-arrest indicate the benefits of ECPR over conventional resuscitation techniques (21% vs. 11%). Moreover, maintaining ECMO after successful resuscitation can offer additional advantages [26–29].

Communication errors can be prevented, enhancing patient safety in high-risk healthcare settings [30]. Acronyms serve as useful guides to prevent communication errors across various medical fields [31]. Around 60–70% of high-risk situation errors result from "human factors" [32]. CALL TO ECLS was developed to reduce communication errors and streamline the qualification process for ECPR by pre-hospital medical teams. Medical personnel can be trained to use the clear information provided in our acronym. The use of standardized tools can balance communication styles among different healthcare professionals and minimize critical intervention response times, such as ECPR [33–35].

Regarding the first version of the protocol, I-CVI and S-CVI-AVE values for importance and relevance, coupled with strong conceptual and developmental frameworks, indicate the high content validity of the criteria and protocol. However, I-CVI values for clarity and unambiguity suggest some criteria revision. The S-CVI-AVE indices for clarity and unambiguity demonstrate acceptable content validity of the protocol. While the S-CVI-UA values did not meet acceptability criteria, this coefficient is sensitive to expert numbers. Given the study's sample size of 35 experts, S-CVI-UA should be treated as additional information. In this case, S-CVI-AVE is recommended. The use of the CVI index is preferred due to its advantages over other indices. However, one weakness of the CVI index is its lack of correction for chance agreement; thus, modified Kappa statistics are recommended. Nevertheless, in this study, due to a large expert sample [34], the chance agreement was close to zero and therefore the modified Kappa was very close to the reported I-CVI.

8. Limitations

The study presents an evaluation of the CALL TO ECLS acronym and is merely a proposal for a quick communication tool. It includes the necessary information about the patient that must be conveyed to qualify the patient for the ECPR procedure. However, qualification criteria may vary between countries, which may necessitate modifications to the acronym. Another limitation of the study is the small number of survey responses, caused by the still limited prevalence of this procedure both in Poland and Europe.

9. Conclusions

It has been shown that the CALL TO ECLS acronym, according to experts, is accurate and contains the necessary content, and can serve as a system to facilitate communication between the pre-hospital environment and specialized units responsible for qualifying patients for the ECPR procedure. Our acronym will not only assist in practical patient handovers in prehospital settings, but will also be useful for the academic community during medical simulations. It includes all the necessary elements that students will need to convey during simulations to qualify a patient for ECPR.

Author Contributions: T.S.: Conceptualization, data curation, writing—original draft preparation. M.P. (Mateusz Putowski): conceptualization, data curation, writing—original draft preparation. M.D.: visualization, investigation A.K.: visualization, investigation. K.Z. supervision, methodology. A.M. software, validation, writing—reviewing and editing. M.P. (Mateusz Puślecki): writing—reviewing and editing. All authors have read and agreed to the published version of the manuscript.

Funding: This research received no external funding from Jagiellonian University Medical College.

Institutional Review Board Statement: Not applicable.

Informed Consent Statement: Not applicable.

Data Availability Statement: The original contributions presented in the study are included in the article, further inquiries can be directed to the corresponding author.

Conflicts of Interest: The authors declare no conflicts of interest.

References

1. Berdowski, J.; Berg, R.A.; Tijssen, J.G.; Koster, R.W. Global incidences of out-of-hospital cardiac arrest and survival rates: Systematic review of 67 prospective. *Resuscitation* **2010**, *81*, 1479–1487. [CrossRef] [PubMed]
2. Grunau, B.; Reynolds, J.; Scheuermeyer, F.; Stenstom, R.; Stub, D.; Pennington, S.; Cheskes, S.; Ramanathan, K.; Christenson, J. Relationship between time-to-ROSC and survival in out-of-hospital cardiac arrest ECPR candidates: When is best time to consider transport to hospital? *Prehosp. Emerg. Care* **2016**, *20*, 615–622. [CrossRef] [PubMed]
3. Monsieurs, K.G.; Nolan, J.P.; Bossaert, L.L.; Greif, R.; Maconochie, I.K.; Nikolaou, N.I.; Perkins, G.D.; Soar, J.; Truhlář, A.; Wyllie, J.; et al. European Resuscitation Council Guidelines for Resuscitation 2015: Section 1. Executive summary. *Resuscitation* **2015**, *95*, 1–80. [CrossRef] [PubMed]
4. Soar, J.; Böttiger, B.W.; Carli, P.; Couper, K.; Deakin, C.D.; Djärv, T.; Lott, C.; Olasveengen, T.; Paal, P.; Pellis, T.; et al. European Resuscitation Council Guidelines 2021: Adult advanced life support. *Resuscitation* **2021**, *161*, 115–151, Erratum in *Resuscitation* **2021**, *167*, 105–106. [CrossRef] [PubMed]
5. Dennis, M.; Lal, S.; Forrest, P.; Nichol, A.; Lamhaut, L.; Totaro, R.J.; Burns, B.; Sandroni, C. In-Depth Extracorporeal Cardiopulmonary Resuscitation in Adult Out-of-Hospital Cardiac Arrest. *J. Am. Heart Assoc.* **2020**, *9*, e016521. [CrossRef] [PubMed] [PubMed Central]
6. Belohlavek, J.; Kucera, K.; Jarkovsky, J.; Franek, O.; Pokorna, M.; Danda, J.; Skripsky, R.; Kandrnal, V.; Balik, M.; Kunstyr, J.; et al. Hyperinvasive approach to out-of hospital cardiac arrest using mechanical chest compression device, prehospital intraarrest cooling, extracorporeal life support and early invasive assessment compared to standard of care. *J. Transl. Med.* **2012**, *10*, 163. [CrossRef] [PubMed] [PubMed Central]
7. Baggs, J.G.; Schmitt, M.H.; Mushlin, A.I.; Mitchell, P.H.; Eldredge, D.H.; Oakes, D.; Hutson, A.D. Association between nurse-physician collaboration and patient outcomes in three intensive care units. *Crit. Care Med.* **1999**, *27*, 1991–1998. [CrossRef] [PubMed]
8. Reader, T.; Flin, R.; Lauche, K.; Cuthbertson, B.H. Non-technical skills in the intensive care unit. *Br. J. Anaesth.* **2006**, *96*, 551–559. [CrossRef] [PubMed]
9. Reader, T.W.; Flin, R.; Mearns, K.; Cuthbertson, B.H. Interdisciplinary communication in the intensive care unit. *Br. J. Anaesth.* **2007**, *98*, 347–352. [CrossRef]
10. Burley, D. Better communication in the emergency department. *Emerg. Nurse* **2011**, *19*, 32–36. [CrossRef]
11. Velji, K.; Baker, G.R.; Fancott, C.; Andreoli, A.; Boaro, N.; Tardif, G.; Aimone, E.; Sinclair, L. Effectiveness of an Adapted SBAR Communication Tool for a Rehabilitation Setting. *Healthc. Q.* **2008**, *11*, 72–79. [CrossRef]
12. Müller, M.; Jürgens, J.; Redaèlli, M.; Klingberg, K.; Hautz, W.E.; Stock, S. Impact of the communication and patient hand-off tool SBAR on patient safety: A systematic review. *BMJ Open* **2018**, *8*, e022202. [CrossRef] [PubMed] [PubMed Central]
13. Dickinson, E.; Limmer, D.; O'Keefe, M.F.; Grant, H.D.; Murray, B. *Emergency Care*, 11th ed.; Prentice Hall: Englewood Cliffs, NJ, USA, 2008; p. 242. ISBN 0-13-500524-8.
14. Polit, D.F.; Beck, C.T.; Owen, S.V. Is the CVI an acceptable indicator of content validity? Appraisal and recommendations. *Res. Nurs. Health* **2007**, *30*, 459–467. [CrossRef] [PubMed]
15. Jeong, W.J.; Lee, J.W.; Yoo, Y.H.; Ryu, S.; Cho, S.W.; Song, K.H.; Park, S.I. Extracorporeal cardiopulmonary resuscitation in bedside echocardiography-diagnosed massive pulmonary embolism. *Am. J. Emerg. Med.* **2015**, *33*, 1545.e1–2. [CrossRef] [PubMed]
16. Morita, S.; Inokuchi, S.; Yamagiwa, T.; Iizuka, S.; Yamamoto, R.; Aoki, H.; Okada, M. Efficacy of portable and percutaneous cardiopulmonary bypass rewarming versus that of conventional internal rewarming for patients with accidental deep hypothermia. *Crit. Care Med.* **2011**, *39*, 1064–1068. [CrossRef]
17. Nakashima, T.; Noguchi, T.; Tahara, Y.; Nishimura, K.; Ogata, S.; Yasuda, S.; Onozuka, D.; Morimura, N.; Nagao, K.; Gaieski, D.F.; et al. Patients with Refractory Out-of-Cardiac Arrest and Sustained Ventricular Fibrillation as Candidates for Extracorporeal Cardiopulmonary Resuscitation—Prospective Multi-Center Observational Study. *Circ. J.* **2019**, *83*, 1011–1018. [CrossRef]
18. Chen, Y.S.; Lin, J.W.; Yu, H.Y.; Ko, W.J.; Jerng, J.S.; Chang, W.T.; Chen, W.J.; Huang, S.C.; Chi, N.H.; Wang, C.H.; et al. Cardiopulmonary resuscitation with assisted extracorporeal life-support versus conventional cardiopulmonary resuscitation in adults with in-hospital cardiac arrest: An observational study and propensity analysis. *Lancet* **2008**, *372*, 554–561. [CrossRef] [PubMed]
19. Lamhaut, L.; Hutin, A.; Puymirat, E.; Jouan, J.; Raphalen, J.H.; Jouffroy, R.; Jaffry, M.; Dagron, C.; An, K.; Dumas, F.; et al. A pre-hospital extracorporeal cardio pulmonary resuscitation (ECPR) strategy for treatment of refractory out hospital cardiac arrest: An observational study and propensity analysis. *Resuscitation* **2017**, *117*, 109–117. [CrossRef]

20. Stub, D.; Bernard, S.; Pellegrino, V.; Smith, K.; Walker, T.; Sheldrake, J.; Hockings, L.; Shaw, J.; Duffy, S.J.; Burrell, A.; et al. Refractory cardiac arrest treated with mechanical CPR, hypothermia, ECMO and early reperfusion (the CHEER trial). *Resuscitation* **2015**, *86*, 88–94. [CrossRef]
21. Kuroki, N.; Abe, D.; Iwama, T.; Suzuki, K.; Sugiyama, K.; Akashi, A.; Hamabe, Y.; Aonuma, K.; Sato, A. Association between delay to coronary reperfusion and outcome in patients with acute coronary syndrome undergoing extracorporeal cardiopulmonary resuscitation. *Resuscitation* **2017**, *114*, 1–6. [CrossRef]
22. Link, M.S.; Berkow, L.C.; Kudenchuk, P.J.; Halperin, H.R.; Hess, E.P.; Moitra, V.K.; Neumar, R.W. Część 7: Adult Advanced Cardiovascular Life Support: 2015 American Heart Association Guidelines Update for Cardiopulmonary Resuscitation and Emergency Cardiovascular Care. *Circulation* **2015**, *132* (Suppl. S2), S444–S464. [CrossRef] [PubMed]
23. Richardson, A.S.C.; Tonna, J.E.; Nanjayya, V.; Nixon, P.; Abrams, D.C.; Raman, L.; Bernard, S.; Finney, S.J.; Grunau, B.; Youngquist, S.T.; et al. Extracorporeal Cardiopulmonary Resuscitation in Adults. Interim Guideline Consensus Statement From the Extracorporeal Life Support Organization. *ASAIO J.* **2021**, *67*, 221–228. [CrossRef] [PubMed]
24. Sip, M.; Puślecki, M.; Kłosiewicz, T.; Zalewski, R.; Dąbrowski, M.; Ligowski, M.; Goszczyńska, E.; Paprocki, C.; Grygier, M.; Lesiak, M.; et al. A concept for the development of a pioneer regional Out-of-Hospital Cardiac Arrest Program to improve patient outcomes. *Kardiol. Pol.* **2020**, *78*, 875–881. [CrossRef]
25. Haas, N.L.; Coute, R.A.; Hsu, C.H.; Cranford, J.A.; Neumar, R.W. Descriptive analysis of extracorporeal cardiopulmonary resuscitation following out-of-hospital cardiac arrest-An ELSO registry study. *Resuscitation* **2017**, *119*, 56–62. [CrossRef]
26. Chan, M.L.; Spertus, J.A.; Tang, F.; Jayaram, N.; Chan, P.S. Missed opportunities in use of Medical Emergency Teams prior to In-Hospital Cardiac Arrest. *Am. Heart J.* **2016**, *177*, 87–95. [CrossRef] [PubMed]
27. American Heart Association. *Advanced Cardiovascular Life Support: Provider Manual*; American Heart Association: Dallas, TX, USA, 2016.
28. Patricio, D.; Peluso, L.; Brasseur, A.; Lheureux, O.; Belliato, M.; Vincent, J.-L.; Creteur, J.; Taccone, F.S. Comparison of extracorporeal and conventional cardiopulmonary resuscitation: A retrospective propensity score matched study. *Crit. Care* **2019**, *23*, 27. [CrossRef] [PubMed]
29. Gao, S.; Liu, G.; Yan, S.; Lou, S.; Gao, G.; Hu, Q.; Zhang, Q.; Qi, J.; Yan, W.; Wang, Q.; et al. Outcomes from adult veno-arterial extracorporeal membrane oxygenation in a cardiovascular disease center from 2009 to 2019. *Perfusion* **2022**, *37*, 235–241. [CrossRef] [PubMed]
30. Vilensky, D.; MacDonald, R.D. Communication errors in dispatch of air medical transport. *Prehosp. Emerg. Care* **2011**, *15*, 39–43. [CrossRef] [PubMed]
31. Yoes, T. Preventing medication errors: Acronyms as strategies. *Okla. Nurse* **2012**, *57*, 15.
32. Kersten, C.; Fink, K.; Michels, G.; Busch, H.J. Crew Resource Management im Schockraum [Crew resource management in emergency centers]. *Med. Klin. Intensivmed. Notfmed.* **2021**, *116*, 377–388, Erratum in *Med. Klin. Intensivmed. Notfmed.* **2021**, *116*, 389. [CrossRef]
33. Turkoski, B.B. Improving patient safety by improving medication communication. *Orthop. Nurs.* **2009**, *28*, 150–154. [CrossRef] [PubMed]
34. Bogenstätter, Y.; Tschan, F.; Semmer, N.K.; Spychiger, M.; Breuer, M.; Marsch, S. How accurate is information transmitted to medical professionals joining a medical emergency? A simulator study. *Hum. Factors* **2009**, *51*, 115–125. [CrossRef] [PubMed]
35. Leonard, M.; Graham, S.; Bonacum, D. The human factor: The critical importance of effective teamwork and communication in providing safe care. *Qual. Saf. Health Care* **2004**, *13* (Suppl. S1), i85–i90. [CrossRef] [PubMed] [PubMed Central]

healthcare

MDPI

Case Report

Successful Intraosseous (IO) Adenosine Administration for the Termination of Supraventricular Tachycardia (SVT) in a 3.5-Year-Old Child—Case Report and Literature Review

Jakub Zachaj [1,*], Łukasz Kręglicki [2,3], Tomasz Sikora [2,4], Katarzyna Moorthi [2,5], Filip Jaśkiewicz [6], Klaudiusz Nadolny [7] and Robert Gałązkowski [1]

1 Medical Emergency Department, Medical University of Warsaw, Litewska 14/16, 00-575 Warsaw, Poland; robert.galazkowski@wum.edu.pl
2 Polish Medical Air Rescue, Księżycowa 5, 01-934 Warsaw, Poland; l.kreglicki@lpr.com.pl (Ł.K.); t.sikora@lpr.com.pl (T.S.); k.moorthi@lpr.com.pl (K.M.)
3 Department of Emergency Medicine, Jagiellonian University Medical College, Michałowskiego 12, 31-126 Cracow, Poland
4 Department of Emergency Medicine, Faculty of Medical Sciences in Katowice, Medical University of Silesia, Poniatowskiego 15, 40-055 Katowice, Poland
5 Military Medical Institute, National Research Institute, Szaserów 128, 04-141 Warsaw, Poland
6 Emergency Medicine and Disaster Medicine Department, Medical University of Lodz, Pomorska 125, 90-419 Lodz, Poland; filip.jaskiewicz@umed.lodz.pl
7 Faculty of Medicine, Department of Emergency Medical Service, Silesian Academy in Katowice, ul. Rolna 43, 40-555 Katowice, Poland; klaudiusz.nadolny@akademiaslaska.pl
* Correspondence: jakub.zachaj@wum.edu.pl

Abstract: Paediatric supraventricular tachycardia (SVT) is a common arrhythmia of great clinical significance. If not treated promptly, it can cause heart failure and cardiogenic shock. Depending on the patient's condition, SVT treatment involves vagal manoeuvres, pharmacological, or direct current cardioversion. The goal of acute SVT management is to immediately convert SVT to a normal sinus rhythm (NSR) and prevent its recurrence. Adenosine is recommended as the first-line treatment for stable SVT by the European Resuscitation Council (ERC) and American Heart Association (AHA) guidelines, when vagal manoeuvres have proven ineffective. The ERC and AHA guidelines recommend the intravenous route of administration. The intraosseous (IO) administration technique is also possible, but still relatively unknown. The aim of this paper is to describe a 3.5-year-old child with SVT that was converted to NSR following IO administration of adenosine. Successful conversion was achieved after the second attempt with the adenosine dose. In the described case, there was no recurrence of SVT.

Keywords: supraventricular tachycardia; intraosseous; adenosine; emergency; paediatrics

1. Introduction

Supraventricular tachycardia (SVT) is the most common cardiac arrythmia among paediatric populations, affecting 1 in 250 to 1000 children [1]. SVT is defined as a rapid and regular heart rate, often exceeding 180 beats per minute (bpm) in children, and 220 bpm in infants. SVT originates above the His bundle [2]. SVT is a broad group of tachyarrhythmias that includes atrioventricular (AV) node-dependant tachyarrhythmias, such as accessory pathway-mediated atrioventricular reciprocating tachycardia (AVRT), as well as atrial tachycardias such as atrial fibrillation, atrial flutter, and ectopic atrial tachycardia [3]. In the case of supraventricular arrhythmias of focal origin, the cause is pathological (increased) automaticity of a specific group of cardiomyocytes or the so-called triggered activity, i.e., early or late depolarization of cardiomyocytes. An alternative mechanism of arrhythmia development is the macro-re-entry mechanism, i.e., the circulation of a depolarization wave stimulating previously depolarized areas that have already regained excitability. Focal arrhythmias caused by increased automaticity or triggered activity are also referred to as non-re-entrant. Focal arrhythmias also include arrhythmias occurring in the micro-re-entry mechanism (short re-entry loop) [4].

The management of SVT depends on the patient's condition [5]. For patients in stable clinical condition with SVT, treatment includes vagal manoeuvres, followed by adenosine if the vagal manoeuvres fail to convert SVT to NSR. Patients in unstable clinical condition with SVT are treated with electrical cardioversion. Adenosine is not effective in the treatment of atrial flutter, atrial fibrillation, and ventricular tachycardia; however, there are rare types of ventricular tachycardias that are adenosine-sensitive (idiopathic VT).

In infants, the signs and symptoms of SVT may be nonspecific and include symptoms such as poor feeding, vomiting, diaphoresis, hypersomnia, and irritability. Toddlers and school-aged children may present with classic cardiac symptoms such as palpations, chest pain, shortness of breath, and syncope. Adolescents may present with this constellation of symptoms, accompanied by anxiety and decreased exercise tolerance. Before initiating appropriate SVT management, factors such as exertion, anxiety, stress, pain, respiratory failure, fever, infections, sepsis, hypoglycaemia, poisoning, hypovolemia, pulmonary embolism, anaphylaxis, anaemia, etc., must be ruled out [6].

2. Case Report

The Helicopter Emergency Services (HEMS) was dispatched to a 3.5-year-old child with arrhythmia. The ground Emergency Medical Team (EMS) on site requested support for patient management and securing their transport to a specialist centre. Once they arrived at the HEMS landing site by ambulance, the patient was lying on a stretcher, was verbally responsive (AVPU), drowsy, and breathing on their own at a rate of approximately 30 breaths per minute on passive oxygen therapy (straight mask) with a flow of 5 litres per minute. The pulse, palpated at the carotid artery, was approximately 200 beats per minute. No monitoring or IV access was established. In a repeated assessment, the patient remained verbally responsive (AVPU—V), the airways were patent and not at risk; there were no secretions in the nasal cavity or oral cavity; respiration was efficient at 24 breaths per minute; there was no shortness of breath or respiratory effort and no central cyanosis; there was slight cyanosis on the periphery (phalanges); SpO_2 was 81–85% (HEMS increased oxygen flow to 10 L/min); auscultatory vesicular murmur was symmetrical bilaterally. SVT with approximately 235 bpm was diagnosed (the ECG recording, on the basis of which SVT was diagnosed, was sent in paper form along with the patient to the hospital, it was not possible to restore the recording from the ground ambulance device's memory); NBP was 144/88; capillary refill was normal; GCS was 12 (E-4, V-4, M-5); glycemia was normal; pupils were equal and reactive to light; there were no meningeal symptoms, convulsions, visible injuries or skin lesions; and the temperature was normal. According to the information provided by the mother, the child had cardiological problems (the child's guardian was unable to determine what diseases the child was suffering from because he was under the influence of alcohol and strong emotional disturbances) and was treated at a specialist clinic. For about 40 min, the child presented with a very rapid heart rate, was crying at first, and was then apathetic. During the ABCDE examination, two attempts to establish peripheral vascular access were unsuccessful. Due to the distance from the specialist centre and air transport conditions (limited space and no possibility of performing some procedures during the flight), and after consultation with the specialist centre, a decision was made to try to stabilize the patient on site. For this purpose, IO access was established by means of the EZ-IO system [Teleflex Medical Triangle Park, NC] with a 15 mm needle inserted into the right tibia near the tibial tuberosity. Once IO access was confirmed, 5 mL of 0.9% NaCl was administered first, followed by lidocaine 2% at a dose of 0.5 mg/kg body weight (8 mg IO). As this failed to alleviate the patient's pain, a second dose of lidocaine 2% was administered, constituting 1/2 of the first dose (4 mg IO). Adenosine was then prepared at a dose of 0.1 mg/kg body weight (1.5 mg), which was administered at 12:59

(the event was recorded in the attached heart monitor tracing). The technique used to deliver adenosine at the scene was the double-syringe technique [DST] (Figure 1). The rhythm temporarily went from 233 bpm to 203 bpm. At 13:05, a decision was made to administer the second dose of 0.2 mg/kg body weight (3 mg) of adenosine. At the next monitoring interval (2 min), the heart rate was 143 bpm; after another 10 min, the patient's heart rate normalized (to 128 bpm) (Figure 2). In both administrations, the adenosine was not diluted. For faster administration, a fluid bolus of 5 mL of 0.9% NaCl was then pushed. After reassessing the patient's condition, the patient was transferred from the ambulance to the helicopter. During transport, the patient was stable, with no recurrence of SVT. The patient was transferred in a good general condition to the staff at the Hospital Emergency Department (ED).

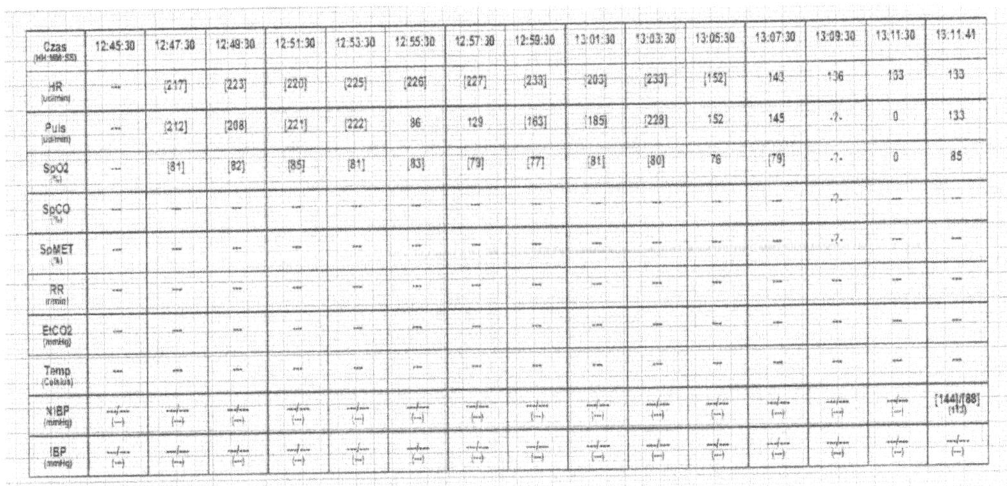

Czas (HH:MM:SS)	12:45:30	12:47:30	12:49:30	12:51:30	12:53:30	12:55:30	12:57:30	12:59:30	13:01:30	13:03:30	13:05:30	13:07:30	13:09:30	13:11:30	13:11:41
HR (ud/min)	---	[217]	[223]	[220]	[225]	[226]	[227]	[233]	[203]	[233]	[152]	143	136	133	133
Puls (ud/min)	---	[212]	[208]	[221]	[222]	86	129	[163]	[185]	[228]	152	145	-?-	0	133
SpO2 (%)	---	[81]	[82]	[85]	[81]	[83]	[79]	[77]	[81]	[80]	76	[79]	-?-	0	85
SpCO (%)	---	---	---	---	---	---	---	---	---	---	---	---	-?-	---	---
SpMET (%)	---	---	---	---	---	---	---	---	---	---	---	---	-?-	---	---
RR (r/min)	---	---	---	---	---	---	---	---	---	---	---	---	---	---	---
EtCO2 (mmHg)	---	---	---	---	---	---	---	---	---	---	---	---	---	---	---
Temp (Celsius)	---	---	---	---	---	---	---	---	---	---	---	---	---	---	---
NIBP (mmHg)	---/--- (---)	---/--- (---)	---/--- (---)	---/--- (---)	---/--- (---)	---/--- (---)	---/--- (---)	---/--- (---)	---/--- (---)	---/--- (---)	---/--- (---)	---/--- (---)	---/--- (---)	---/--- (---)	[144]/[88] (113)
IBP (mmHg)	---/--- (---)	---/--- (---)	---/--- (---)	---/--- (---)	---/--- (---)	---/--- (---)	---/--- (---)	---/--- (---)	---/--- (---)	---/--- (---)	---/--- (---)	---/--- (---)	---/--- (---)	---/--- (---)	---/--- (---)

Figure 1. First recording of heart rate and reaction to the first dose of adenosine (Defiguard Touch 7, Schiller Schweiz AG, Bachstrasse 30, 8912 Obfelden, Switzerland). Asterisks means that no blood pressure measurement was taken during the given interval.

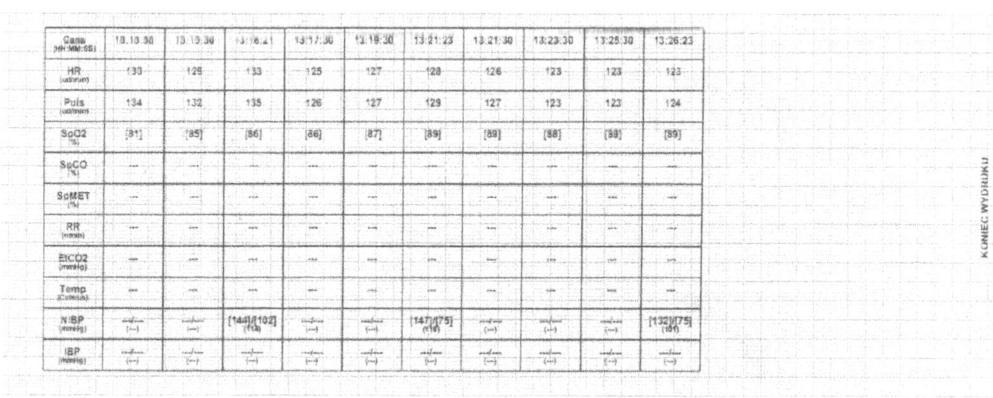

Czas (HH:MM:SS)	13:13:30	13:15:30	13:16:21	13:17:30	13:19:30	13:21:23	13:21:30	13:23:30	13:25:30	13:26:23
HR (ud/min)	130	129	133	125	127	128	126	123	123	123
Puls (ud/min)	134	132	135	126	127	129	127	123	123	124
SpO2 (%)	[81]	[85]	[86]	[86]	[87]	[89]	[89]	[88]	[88]	[89]
SpCO (%)	---	---	---	---	---	---	---	---	---	---
SpMET (%)	---	---	---	---	---	---	---	---	---	---
RR (r/min)	---	---	---	---	---	---	---	---	---	---
EtCO2 (mmHg)	---	---	---	---	---	---	---	---	---	---
Temp (Celsius)	---	---	---	---	---	---	---	---	---	---
NIBP (mmHg)	---/--- (---)	---/--- (---)	[144]/[102] ([illegible])	---/--- (---)	---/--- (---)	[147]/[75] ([illegible])	---/--- (---)	---/--- (---)	---/--- (---)	[132]/[75] ([illegible])
IBP (mmHg)	---/--- (---)	---/--- (---)	---/--- (---)	---/--- (---)	---/--- (---)	---/--- (---)	---/--- (---)	---/--- (---)	---/--- (---)	---/--- (---)

Figure 2. Second recording of heart rate and reaction to the second dose of adenosine (Defiguard Touch 7, Schiller Schweiz AG, Bachstrasse 30, 8912 Obfelden, Switzerland). Asterisks means that no blood pressure measurement was taken during the given interval.

3. Discussion

As mentioned previously, the choice of SVT management depends on the patient's hemodynamic and clinical condition (patients in stable clinical condition with SVT vs. patients in unstable clinical condition with SVT). Clinical findings in SVT may differ, depending on the age of the child and the duration of SVT. ERC and AHA guidelines recommend vagal manoeuvres and adenosine as the first-line treatment for stable SVT [7,8].

Adenosine can serve as a diagnostic or therapeutic agent. In diagnostics, adenosine is used in myocardial perfusion stress imaging by virtue of its vasodilatory effects. In a therapeutic setting, adenosine is used for its antiarrhythmic properties in supraventricular tachycardia and can function as a diagnostic tool, depending on the type of SVT, in both paediatric and adult patients [9]. Adenosine can also unmask (though not terminate) atrial flutter in cases of unclear tachycardia, if used for diagnostic issues. Adenosine is indicated as an adjunct to thallium-201 in myocardial perfusion scintigraphy, as well as for the conversion of paroxysmal supraventricular tachycardia into sinus rhythm. Adenosine has a short duration of action (half-life <10 s) and a wide therapeutic window [10]. Agonism of adenosine receptors A1 and A2 reduces conduction time in the atrioventricular node of the heart. Conduction velocity is decreased by inducing potassium efflux and inhibiting calcium influx through channels in the nerve cells, leading to hyperpolarization and an increased threshold for calcium-dependent action potentials. The decreased conduction time leads to an antiarrhythmic effect. Adenosine has an effect on the cells of the AV node. Due to its effect on the AV node, Adenosine can only terminate re-entrant SVT involving the AV node in the re-entry circuit (AVRT and AVNRT) but not in cases of intra-atrial re-entry or focal atrial tachycardia. The inhibition of calcium influx reduces the activity of adenylate cyclase, relaxing the vascular smooth muscles. Relaxed vascular smooth muscles lead to increased blood flow through normal coronary arteries but not through stenotic arteries, allowing for the easier uptake of thallium-201 in normal coronary arteries [10,11]. The most frequently described side effects of adenosine administration are bronchoconstriction, seizures, and hypersensitivity. Adenosine can also cause bradycardia, leading to *torsade de pointes*, especially in patients with a prolonged QT interval. A total of six cases of arrhythmia caused by the administration of adenosine in paediatric patients (aged 0–16 years with overt or hidden Wolf–Parkinson–White syndrome [WPW]) have been described in the literature. The cases mentioned included three cases of atrial fibrillation, two cases of atrial flutter and one case of ventricular fibrillation. In three cases, the arrhythmias resolved spontaneously, while in the remaining cases they required treatment with amiodarone or amiodarone administration and electrical cardioversion [12]. Patients with an overdose of adenosine may present with asystole, heart block, or cardiac ischemia. These effects are generally short-lived. Patients with an overdose should receive symptomatic and supportive care, which may include a slow intravenous injection of theophylline [9,10].

Adenosine failure occurs when its administration does not result in a definitive or sustained termination of tachycardia. There are three scenarios that cause this, as follows: administration errors (e.g., insufficient adenosine dose), failure to terminate the arrhythmia, and insufficient duration of the adenosine effect [13].

Adenosine should be administered into a venous vessel as close as possible to the heart (vein in the antecubital bend). Regardless of the choice of procedure (pharmacologic or electrical cardioversion), the patient must be fully monitored, and the team must be ready to start advanced life-saving procedures. The literature describes two administration techniques. Standard guidelines recommended adenosine to be administered IV with an immediate bolus of normal saline solution (NSS; double-syringe technique [DST]). Only one syringe is used as part of the second technique (single-syringe technique [SST]). In this technique, adenosine is diluted with NSS. SST may be as safe as DST, equally effective for SVT termination, or even potentially more effective with the first dose. SST constitutes a simpler and more rapid approach, obviating the need for syringe-switching or using a three-way stopcock, which was actually used to administer the drug in the described case, resulting in a reduction in the margin of error in adenosine administration [14,15]. In the described case, DST was used. The literature formulates no recommendations regarding the selection of an adenosine delivery technique when intraosseous access is used by the rescuers.

The IO technique has presented itself as a possible route of adenosine administration. It is fast, reliable, requires minimal training, and can be implemented rapidly. This technique is recommended by AHA guidelines [7]. ERC indicates intravenous administration as the preferred method of adenosine administration (there is insufficient evidence supporting effective and safe IO adenosine administration) [8]. The ERC indicates exactly when intraosseous access should be performed as part of Paediatric Advanced Life Support (PALS). An attempt to establish intraosseous access should be made when the chances of obtaining peripheral access are low and already at an early stage of treatment (alternative access) [7]. Multiple studies have shown the importance and reliability of IO access in the paediatric population [16]. IO access refers to the placement a specialized hollow-bore needle through the cortex of a bone into the medullary space for infusion or for collecting laboratory samples (before submitting the sample for laboratory testing, it must be properly marked). The distal femur, proximal tibia, and distal tibia are recommended sites for IO placement in neonates and children. The preferred access site in infants and children is the anteromedial surface of the tibia, approximately 1 to 2 cm below the tibia tuberosity [17]. The choice of where to perform intraosseous access depends mainly on the device used. It seems reasonable to assume that access, as in the case of venous access, should be performed as close to the heart as possible (humeral head) due to the short half-life of adenosine in the bloodstream. However, obtaining such access will depend on the device available. Currently, pre-hospital emergency services in Poland (emergency medical services, hospital emergency departments, and HEMS) have access to both mechanical and manual devices for IO access. The mechanical devices include NIO-P (New Intraosseous—Pediatric, PerSys Medical, Houston, Tx), BIG-P (Bone Injection Gun—Pediatric, PerSys Medical, Houston, Tx) and Arrow EZ-IO (Teleflex Medical Triangle Park, NC—used by HEMS teams in Poland). Manual devices include the Jamshidi IO needle (Jamshidi, Baxter HealthCare Corporation, Deerfield, Ill) and Cook IO needle (Cook Medical, O'Halloran Road National Technology Park Limerick, Ireland). The mechanical devices used to perform IO access are more reliable, take a shorter amount of time to obtain vascular access, and require less training before they can be used correctly. An important element when selecting a device for intraosseous access is the chance of success in performing this type of access upon the first attempt. Mechanical devices are much more advantageous in this respect [18]. Regardless of whether intraosseous access is performed using a mechanical or manual device, a three-way tap will be an integral part of the access. Its use requires a certain amount of fluid inside, which may affect the therapeutic effect of adenosine, especially when SST is used (too low a drug dose). Performing intraosseous access involves certain risks. The most frequently mentioned adverse events are as follows: failure to enter the bone marrow, with extravasation or subperiosteal infusion; through-and-through penetration of the bone; osteomyelitis (rare in short-term use); physeal plate injury; local infection; skin necrosis; pain; compartment syndrome; and fat and bone microemboli (reported but are rare) [19].

One of the elements of the intraosseous access procedure is proper analgesia. When using the EZ-IO device, the manufacturer recommends 0.5 mL/kg body weight of 2% lidocaine without adrenaline and preservatives in a slow bolus (120 s), followed by 2–5 mL NS push (60 s) [20]. Although lidocaine has antiarrhythmic effects, it is not a pharmacological agent recommended by the AHA and ERC for interrupting an episode of SVT. However, its influence on the condition of the presented patient cannot be ruled out.

In the literature on intraosseous adenosine administration, there is evidence both confirming and rejecting the effectiveness of adenosine administration via this route. In 1994, research was carried out on piglets to demonstrate whether adenosine used IO was effective or not. Conclusions from this research indicated that the intraosseous route is an effective way of administering adenosine. Moreover, the peripheral venous dose required to achieve atrioventricular block is higher than the central venous dose, while the intraosseous dose falls between the central venous and peripheral venous doses of adenosine [21]. The effectiveness of adenosine in terminating supraventricular tachycardia in a paediatric patient was confirmed in the case of an 11-day-old boy described by Friedman (conversion to NSR with 100 mcg of adenosine, an early dose was given prior to attempting cardioversion, a saline flush was not reported) [22]. In 2012, a paper by Goodman and Lu was published, presenting cases of a 2-month-old and a 4-month-old child diagnosed with SVT. In both cases, the administration of adenosine did not achieve the intended result. In the first case, rhythm conversion occurred through the administration of adenosine via intravenous access (250 mcg IO, 100 mcg IV). In the second case, central access was used to administer the drug (200 mcg IO), but with SVT recurrence [5]. The cases described by Friedman and Goodman and Lu were compiled by Clark. Clark stated that intraosseous adenosine does not appear to be as effective as intravenous administration. However, he emphasizes that the reason for the failure of intraosseous administration may be the delivery technique (drug dose, NS bolus rate) [23]. In the following years, papers were published proving the effectiveness of intraosseous adenosine administration. Helleman et al. described the case of a 2-week-old boy who experienced an episode of SVT. Conversion to NSR was achieved with 0.5 mg adenosine, diluted to 3 mL NS (SST technique) [24]. Fidancı et al. reported the case of a 28-day-old boy in whom the conversion of SVT to NSR was achieved with adenosine (3450 g–0.1 mcg of adenosine per kg, single dose) [25]. The described case concerns a child older than 12 months, which makes it unique in the context of the previously described cases.

4. Conclusions

The described case of a paediatric patient with an episode of SVT concerns a hemodynamically unstable patient. Stable patients should be transported to the nearest paediatric cardiology department, even if tachycardia is present (depending as well on local conditions and the scope of practice and experience of the emergency team).

In the presented case report of a 3.5-year-old child, SVT was converted to NSR using two doses of adenosine, administered in accordance with ERC guidelines using the IO route. IO access was established due to difficulties in the cannulation of peripheral vessels and the technical conditions associated with transporting injured persons using a helicopter. The patient was transferred to the emergency room in good general condition.

There is no evidence in the literature that unanimously supports or rejects intraosseous adenosine administration. Further definitive studies are needed to determine whether IO administration of adenosine in stable SVT is safe and effective for paediatric patients. In future studies, special attention should be paid to the technique of intraosseous adenosine administration. It is necessary to determine whether SST or DST is more effective for adenosine administration. It is necessary to determine the recommended site for intraosseous access and the potential impact of lidocaine on the termination of an SVT episode.

Author Contributions: Conceptualization, J.Z. and Ł.K.; methodology, R.G. and K.N.; investigation, J.Z; resources, T.S.; data curation, T.S.; writing—original draft preparation, J.Z. and Ł.K.; writing—review and editing, K.M. and F.J.; supervision, R.G. and K.N.; project administration, J.Z. All authors have read and agreed to the published version of the manuscript.

Funding: This research received no external funding.

Institutional Review Board Statement: Not applicable.

Informed Consent Statement: Informed consent was obtained from all subjects involved in the study.

Data Availability Statement: Data are contained within the article.

Conflicts of Interest: The authors declare no conflicts of interest.

References

1. Brugada, J.; Blom, N.; Sarquella-Brugada, G.; Blomstrom-Lundqvist, C.; Deanfield, J.; Janousek, J.; Abrams, D.; Bauersfeld, U.; Brugada, R.; Drago, F.; et al. Pharmacological and non-pharmacological therapy for arrhythmias in the pediatric population: EHRA and AEPC-Arrhythmia Working Group joint consensus statement. *Europace* **2013**, *15*, 1337–1382. [CrossRef] [PubMed]
2. Richardson, C.; Silver, E.S. Management of Supraventricular Tachycardia in Infants. *Paediatr. Drugs* **2017**, *19*, 539–551. [CrossRef] [PubMed]
3. Ko, J.K.; Deal, B.J.; Strasburger, J.F.; Benson, D. Supraventricular tachycardia mechanisms and their age distribution in pediatric patients. *Am. J. Cardiol.* **1992**, *69*, 1028–1032. [CrossRef] [PubMed]
4. Patel, A.; Markowitz, S.M. Atrial tachycardia: Mechanisms and management. *Expert. Rev. Cardiovasc. Ther.* **2008**, *6*, 811–822. [CrossRef] [PubMed]
5. Goodman, I.S.; Lu, C.J. Intraosseous infusion is unreliable for adenosine delivery in the treatment of supraventricular tachycardia. *Pediatr. Emerg. Care* **2012**, *28*, 47–48. [CrossRef] [PubMed]
6. Schlechte, E.A.; Boramanand, N.; Funk, M. Supraventricular tachycardia in the pediatric primary care setting: Age-related presentation, diagnosis, and management. *J. Pediatr. Health Care* **2008**, *22*, 289–299. [CrossRef] [PubMed]
7. Van de Voorde, P.; Turner, N.M.; Djakow, J.; de Lucas, N.; Martinez-Mejias, A.; Biarent, D.; Bingham, R.; Brissaud, O.; Hoffmann, F.; Johannesdottir, G.B.; et al. European Resuscitation Council Guidelines 2021: Paediatric Life Support. *Resuscitation* **2021**, *161*, 327–387. [CrossRef] [PubMed]
8. Topjian, A.A.; Raymond, T.T.; Atkins, D.; Chan, M.; Duff, J.P.; Jr, B.L.J.; Lasa, J.J.; Lavonas, E.J.; Levy, A.; Mahgoub, M.; et al. Pediatric Basic and Advanced Life Support: 2020 American Heart Association Guidelines for Cardiopulmonary Resuscitation and Emergency Cardiovascular Care. *Circulation* **2020**, *142* (Suppl. S2), S469–S523. [CrossRef] [PubMed]
9. Singh, S.; McKintosh, R. Adenosine. In *StatPearls [Internet]*; StatPearls Publishing: Treasure Island, FL, USA, 2023. Available online: https://www.ncbi.nlm.nih.gov/books/NBK519049/ (accessed on 28 August 2023).
10. Available online: https://www.accessdata.fda.gov/drugsatfda_docs/label/2014/020059s017s018lbl.pdf (accessed on 13 January 2023).
11. Zoghbi, G.J.; Iskandrian, A.E. Selective adenosine agonists and myocardial perfusion imaging. *J. Nucl. Cardiol.* **2012**, *19*, 126–141. [CrossRef] [PubMed]
12. Available online: https://rejestry.ezdrowie.gov.pl/api/rpl/medicinal-products/298/characteristic (accessed on 25 July 2024).
13. Shortland, J.; Saravu Vijayashankar, S.; Sanatani, S. When Adenosine Does Not Work: Apparent and Real Adenosine-Resistant Tachycardia. *Pediatr. Emerg. Care* **2022**, *38*, 235–240. [CrossRef] [PubMed]
14. Kotruchin, P.; Chaiyakhan, I.; Kamonsri, P.; Chantapoh, W.; Serewiwattana, N.; Kaweenattayanon, N.; Narangsiya, N.; Lorcharassriwong, P.; Korsakul, K.; Thawepornpuriphong, P.; et al. Comparison between the double-syringe and the single-syringe techniques of adenosine administration for terminating supraventricular tachycardia: A pilot, randomized controlled trial. *Clin. Cardiol.* **2022**, *45*, 583–589. [CrossRef] [PubMed] [PubMed Central]
15. Miyawaki, I.A.; Gomes, C.; Moreira, V.C.S.; Marques, I.R.; de Souza, I.A.F.; Silva, C.H.A.; Júnior, J.E.R.L.; Huh, K.; McDowell, M.; Padrao, E.M.H.; et al. The Single-Syringe Versus the Double-Syringe Techniques of Adenosine Administration for Supraventricular Tachycardia: A Systematic Review and Meta-Analysis. *Am. J. Cardiovasc. Drugs* **2023**, *23*, 341–353. [CrossRef] [PubMed]
16. Tobias, J.D.; Ross, A.K. Intraosseous infusions: A review for the anesthesiologist with a focus on pediatric use. *Anesth. Analg.* **2010**, *110*, 391–401. [CrossRef] [PubMed]
17. Dornhofer, P.; Kellar, J.Z. Intraosseous Vascular Access 5 June 2023. In *StatPearls [Internet]*; StatPearls Publishing: Treasure Island, FL, USA, 2024. Available online: https://pubmed.ncbi.nlm.nih.gov/32119260/ (accessed on 13 January 2023). [PubMed]
18. Szarpak, L.; Ladny, J.R.; Dabrowski, M.; Ladny, M.; Smereka, J.; Ahuja, S.; Ruetzler, K. Comparison of 4 Pediatric Intraosseous Access Devices: A Randomized Simulation Study. *Pediatr. Emerg. Care* **2020**, *36*, e568–e572. [CrossRef] [PubMed]
19. Available online: https://www.rch.org.au/clinicalguide/guideline_index/intraosseous_access/ (accessed on 23 July 2023).
20. Available online: https://www.teleflex.com/global/clinical-resources/documents/MCI-2019-0394_VA_DS_EZ-IO_Intraosseus_Vascular_Access_LR.pdf (accessed on 13 January 2023).
21. Getschman, S.J.; Dietrich, A.M.; Franklin, W.H.; Allen, H.D. Intraosseous adenosine. As effective as peripheral or central venous administration? *Arch. Pediatr. Adolesc. Med.* **1994**, *148*, 616–619. [CrossRef] [PubMed]
22. Friedman, F.D. Intraosseous adenosine for the termination of supraventricular tachycardia in an infant. *Ann. Emerg. Med.* **1996**, *28*, 356–358. [PubMed]
23. BET 1: Intraosseous adenosine for the termination of paroxysmal supraventricular tachycardia in children. *Emerg. Med. J.* **2014**, *31*, 604–605. [CrossRef] [PubMed]
24. Helleman, K.; Kirpalani, A.; Lim, R. A Novel Method of Intraosseous Infusion of Adenosine for the Treatment of Supraventricular Tachycardia in an Infant. *Pediatr. Emerg. Care* **2017**, *33*, 47–48. [CrossRef] [PubMed]
25. Fidancı, İ.; Güleryüz, O.D.; Yenice, Ö.D. Successful intraosseous adenosine administration in a newborn infant with supraventricular tachycardia. *Turk. J. Pediatr.* **2020**, *62*, 1064–1068. [CrossRef] [PubMed]

healthcare

MDPI

Perspective

"Even Though the System Had Failed Him His Entire Life, We Were Failing Him Yet Again": How Clinical, Welfare, and Penal Medicine Interact to Drive Health Inequities and Medical Moral Injury

Siddhi S. Ganesh [1,*], Kyle B. Joyner [2], Shamsher Samra [3], Ricky N. Bluthenthal [1] and Todd W. Schneberk [2]

1 Department of Population and Public Health Sciences, Keck School of Medicine, University of Southern California, Los Angeles, CA 90032, USA; rbluthen@usc.edu
2 Los Angeles General Medical Center, Department of Emergency Medicine, Keck School of Medicine, University of Southern California, Los Angeles, 1200 N State St, Los Angeles, CA 90033, USA; todd.schneberk@med.usc.edu (T.W.S.); Kyle.joyner@med.usc.edu (K.B.J.)
3 Department of Emergency Medicine, David Geffen School of Medicine, University of California, Los Angeles, CA 90095, USA; sssamra@ucla.edu
* Correspondence: ssganesh@usc.edu

Abstract: Adam, a justice-involved young man, was brought into the emergency department at the county hospital in cardiogenic shock due to a recurring episode of injection-drug-use-related infective endocarditis (IDU-IE). Adam had initiated injection opioid use in prison. He was surgically treated for the previous episodes of IDU-IE but was unable to fully recover due to limitations in care within penal medicine. This case report explores the prison as a determinant of health, interactions between clinical, welfare, and penal medicine' to produce and maintain health inequities, and structural drivers of physician moral injury through an interview with Adam and reflexive writings from emergency medicine physicians. This case demonstrates the need for three types of structural health interventions: (1) restorative justice, community-based reentry programs, and housing as welfare medicine, (2) increased harm reduction services across healthcare, especially penal medicine, and (3) equitable institutional protocols (contrary to ambiguous guidelines) to treat clinical conditions like IDU-IE that disproportionately impact structurally vulnerable patients.

Keywords: substance use disorder; incarceration; medication for opioid use disorder; harm reduction; moral injury

1. Background

Adam had a history of congenital heart disease. He was born with a bicuspid aortic valve, resulting in symptomatic aortic stenosis that was treated surgically in his childhood. Growing up with eight other siblings, when he was ten years old, his stepfather told him he was adopted. Looking back at this major turning point, Adam said the following:

> *"I started acting out...As I got older, it just became a cycle of me getting in and out of jail. And then when I turned 18, I started going to the county jail. And then I started doing time in prison...I had never seen heroin until I went to prison. I caught hep-C in prison...Prison didn't really teach me anything."*

Upon leaving prison, Adam started experiencing opioid withdrawal symptoms and sought illicit market heroin to manage these symptoms. Soon after, he was diagnosed with his first episode of injection-drug-use-related infective endocarditis (IDU-IE) and was treated surgically. However, due to failures in medical care at different carceral facilities, he was not provided with medications to complete his outpatient antibiotic treatment course. Around this time, Adam was diagnosed with deep vein thrombosis (DVT) in his leg and a second episode of IDU-IE. An additional surgery was performed to treat the recurrence of IDU-IE.

Post-surgery and release from prison, Adam looked for substance use treatment programs but was unable to enroll due to delays in medical record transfer requests and program ineligibility due to his complex medical history. This was exacerbated by the insurance transition from his carceral care provision back to Medicaid [1] and the delay in enrollment after application. Adam reinitiated substance use, attributing it to this lack of programs and services. To stop using opioids, he even moved away from his neighborhood and searched for housing programs, to no avail. Eventually, he was arrested and returned to jail due to his drug use. There, he started to feel unwell again.

Obtaining health care while incarcerated included barriers to accessing physicians, inconsistencies in communication between providers, and access to medication. He shared the following:

> *"In the county jail they treat you like they don't care. Everything is like, 'Oh, drink some water you'll be alright, drink some water you'll be alright'. [About the process of seeing a physician] You fill out a form. . .Once you fill out the form, it's 13–14 days just for you to see the doctor. And then. . . It feels kinda hopeless you know. To fill out a form because it's like, 'Oh I have this wrong with me, if I fill out a form, by the time I get there, I'll probably already be OK.' So that's how a lot of people feel like. I might go look for someone who has the pills I need. I went looking for pills for a cold. Even the nurses will give you the medicine because they know it will take forever to see the doctor. It's just such as struggle even just to get anything then and there."*

Adam spent crucial time waiting for a cardiology referral assured to him by one provider and later found out from another provider that he never had a formal referral. In jail, he did not have access to specific analgesic and antibiotic medications prescribed to him at his latest hospital discharge. Adam visited the physician five times prior to being transported to the local hospital for his most recent episode of IDU-IE. The day he was brought into the hospital, he woke up with shortness of breath, collapsed to the ground, and yelled "man down" multiple times before he was brought to the hospital.

In the hospital, Adam was admitted to the cardiology service for heart failure from a third episode of recurrent IDU-IE. His symptoms began with mild shortness of breath and rapidly progressed to cardiogenic shock with multiorgan failure. He was diagnosed with severely complicated endocarditis with a valvular abscess requiring corrective surgery. Adam was denied a third valve surgery due to his history of substance use and died soon after.

Prior to his death, the emergency medicine (EM) physicians caring for Adam called other hospitals to attempt transfer and involved their supervising institution's ethics committee. Limited by his incarcerated status, the physicians were only able to successfully advocate for increased visitation rights to see his mother and partner before his passing. Adam provided written consent to publish the contents of his interview and the physician's submitting reflexive writings. In this interview, he said the following:

> *"I just, I just want a chance. A good, solid chance."*

2. Social Analysis Concepts

The United States incarcerates more people than any other independent democracy, disproportionately disenfranchising people who are African American, Hispanic, and Indigenous [2]. For instance, while 14% of the United States population is African American, they make up 35% of the incarcerated population [3]. Hyper-incarceration refers to this disproportionate incarceration rate and is a form of structural violence [4–6]. Structural violence describes the ways in which large-scale forces (such as racism and immiseration) and inequitable public policies (i.e., restricting public support for low-income people, criminalizing housing insecurity) become embedded within institutions (such as medicine), causing harm to specific individuals and communities [4–6] Within medical institutions, Seim and

DiMario identified three terrains, namely, clinical, welfare, and penal medicine that have focused their interventions on the governing poor [1]. In this case study, we explore these interactions via experiences shared by Adam and his emergency medicine clinicians.

While the United States constitution does not guarantee healthcare, incarcerated people have a right to the community standard of healthcare [2]. However, prisons and jails serve as determinants of health due to various overlapping and intersecting factors. These include exposure to infectious disease, access to treatment, and a paucity of resources for societal reentry to name a few [7]. Adam reported first injecting heroin in prison and continuing to use opioids upon release. IDU-IE is an infection of the heart valve that requires surgery and parenteral antibiotics for 6–8 weeks. People who inject opioids can develop IDU-IE from bacteria entering the bloodstream due to lack of sterile needles or sterile injection supplies, reusing or sharing needles, being injected by others, and substance contamination from lack of safe supply [8–10]. Multi-level barriers to providing Medications for Opioid Use Disorder (MOUD) in criminal justice settings can exacerbate these existing risks [11] Current American Association for Thoracic Surgery (AATS) guidelines on the surgical treatment of infective endocarditis recommend that "normal indications for surgery [should be] applied to people who use drugs (PWUD), but management must include treatment of addiction" [12] However, in Adam's case, he was unable to access MOUD both in criminal justice settings and upon reentry. Beyond that, this case elucidates how substance use treatment extends far beyond MOUD and includes wrap-around services like housing, re-entry, and employment programs.

Emergency departments (EDs) are often referred to as the safety net of the United States healthcare system, as EDs provide medical care to any and all patients regardless of insurance status [1,13,14]. ED's provide care to materially deprived communities [1] and, consequently, EM physicians often take on a bridging role as providers of social emergency medicine [13] This has a profound effect on those practicing in the ED. Concurrently, one metanalysis showed that EM physicians had the highest levels of burnout, as high as 40%, and were more vulnerable to burnout than physicians from other departments [15]. According to the United States Department of Veterans Affairs and the National Center for Post-traumatic Stress Disorder (PTSD), under traumatic, stressful, or unprecedented circumstances, individuals may perpetrate, witness, and/or fail to prevent the occurrence of events that go against moral beliefs or expectations they hold deeply [16]. Moral injury can take place among healthcare workers if and when they have to make difficult decisions when triaging life-and-death cases and/or under circumstances involving resource allocation or when they believe they or the system should have been able to save a patient's life but were not able to do so [16].

Adam's case emphasizes three main social concepts: (1) hyper-incarceration [4] and prison as a determinant of health; (2) interactions between clinical, welfare, and penal medicine [1] to produce and maintain health inequities; and (3) moral injury as a structural phenomenon [16].

2.1. Hyper-Incarceration and Prison Are Determinants of Health

The adverse events in his childhood and subsequent punitive interventions [17,18] facilitated his first injection opioid use in prison. Below, Adam describes the impact of that initiating heroin use in prison and the lack of structural support for substance use disorder (SUD) treatment. In prison, he participated in a computer program for substance use disorders but noted that no other treatment was available. Regarding infective endocarditis, he shared the following:

> *"Then I went to prison again and I found out I had caught. . .endocarditis. And I got the surgery for endocarditis the first time. And after that, I didn't get a chance to recover the right way. I got sent back to jail. I didn't get sent to a program. I didn't get the right transitioning into the life I should have lived. I went straight to jail. And in jail I started doing drugs again. . .[I did not have a] support system to help me fully. [A support system that was not], 'It's my way or the high way', [instead a support system*

that said], 'Here let me help you take a step forward, here let me help you step forward and take a step forward.'" (Adam)

He described the medical treatment he received in prison as follows:

> *"When you guys send forms with us of recommendations and [they state] 'this person is supposed to take this medication, and this medicine and this medicine', when it gets there [i.e., prison], everything gets disregarded, and it goes down the hill. it goes to the doctor and the doctor says. . .Like the last time when I got antibiotics, the doctor told [me], 'Oh, I don't really think you need this.'"* (Adam)

2.2. Clinical, Penal, and Welfare Medicine Interact to Produce and Maintain Patient Health Inequities

Adam's recurrent episodes of IDU-IE were a result of incarceration, lack of access to MOUD, antibiotic treatment discontinuity in prison [19,20], and subsequent inability to recover fully from his previous surgeries. Below, Adam's clinician reflects on the factors that led to a recurrence of endocarditis:

> *"Unfortunately, because of a combination of a lack of treatment follow-through, access to healthcare, and drug abuse programs in prison, Adam had a relapse of his endocarditis."* (One of Adam's physicians)

Adam identified that his social network and neighborhood shaped his opioid use and identified the services that would have supported treatment. He said the following:

> *"My drug addiction was just hard because [of] the people I hang out with, I go back to the same shit you know. That's why I need a program to help me get into housing because when I don't have nowhere to go, I go the hood."*

He moved into to his sister's home in an attempt *"to get away from the environment"*. When asked what prompted his return, he said the following:

> *"I just didn't have no money. So, I went back to where I knew I could get money, you know. . . It was the addiction and the lack of support that I had, I had my sister, but I didn't have nobody else. So, I didn't have anywhere to go, so like fuck it I'll just go back home. I know that there's programs where they take you and they build you and build you until you get home and they provide you with housing, provide with you like a job. Like if I was at my sisters and I had a job, I think I would be able to make it. Like, Suboxone clinics I think."* (Adam)

Adam attempted to get into a program but did not meet the eligibility criteria:

> *"I went through the [recovery] and I tried to go check into a [substance use] program, and I needed to find the right program because that program wouldn't take me due to my medical issues."* (Adam)

Aspects of Adam's case elucidate how institutionalized deservingness [6] in clinical medicine operates via treatment futility and resource rationing [9] against disenfranchised and materially deprived patients [21,22] in this case, resulting in the determination of poor surgical candidacy [23].

> *"...Our surgeon colleagues felt like they could not justifiably offer care to this poor individual due to it being too high risk, a short-term solution, and unfair from a resource standpoint to perform a third surgery."* (One of Adam's physicians)

Here, Adam's physician describes how his structural vulnerabilities (incarcerated status and complex history of recurring IDU-IE) further limited their ability to care for him:

> *"We made phone calls to other hospitals but were limited by his incarcerated status and complex history."* (One of Adam's physicians)

2.3. Medical Moral Injury Is Structurally Driven

In medicine, moral injury via commission occurs when a clinician acts against their beliefs, whereas moral injury via omission takes place when a clinician is unable to act on their deeply held beliefs [16] In times of overlapping public health crises, such the intersection of the opioid mortality crisis, dissolving social safety net, inaccessible wrap-around support, and hyper-incarceration in Adam's case, clinicians may witness what they believe to be unjustifiable/unfair acts or policies that may lead to a feeling of betrayal from individuals, systems, and institutions of power [16]. The reflexive ethnographic writings by Adam's EM clinicians on this case demonstrate how an institutional failure [19] to account for the needs of structurally vulnerable patients [5] displaces that burden onto individual-level clinicians who feel restricted in their ability to provide care:

> *"When his life intersected with ours in healthcare, I feel like he had been failed so many times by society and we did not have the ability to help him."* (One of Adam's physicians)

> *"We had to tell Adam that there was nothing we could do for him. We had to tell him, that even though the system had failed him his entire life, we were failing him yet again, and this time our failures were going to cost him his life."* (One of Adam's physicians)

Such cases are stressful and procedurally ambiguous, and clinicians are constrained by structural vulnerabilities such as incarceration status that do not have clear and equitable guidelines for care. Altogether, these may result in moral injury [16,22].

> *"The case has stuck with me more than any other as a physician because I have never been in the situation of telling a [young patient] that they will die of an illness where we typically do have interventions to offer."* (One of Adam's physicians)

> *"I have question[ed] if I felt like the principle of justice was not honored in his final days. He had self-admittedly made serious mistakes and poor life choices that resulted in him being in this situation. But he also expressed a desire to change, to seek treatment, and to try to turn his life around. He also was born with a congenital condition that predisposed him to this disease, suffered from adverse childhood experiences, and had been in the cycle of incarceration and substance use—these have all been studied in medical and psychological literature to be outside of an individual's control."* (One of Adam's physicians)

3. Discussion

Adam's case emphasizes how structural failures such as hyper-incarceration and punitive justice in the United States result in outcomes that are displaced onto institutions, such as hospitals and medical systems [1,4]. Here, they remain unaddressed due to a lack of bureaucratic protocols and guidelines outlined for incarcerated patients, resource rationing and deservingness, and because of conditions arising from the structural failures themselves. For instance, Adam was declared a poor candidate for surgery due to failures of care in the penal healthcare system, i.e., barriers to medication adherence, MOUD access, and not being able to see a doctor on time [1,8,9,11]. Within medicine, the downstream impacts of institutional failures are displaced onto frontline workers, including physicians, nurses, social workers, social services workers, and program coordinators, who attempt to navigate medical systems alongside structurally vulnerable patients [1,5]. At this point, frontline workers face barriers to access, care, and treatment from policy failures that are far beyond their clinical scope. In Adam's case, clinicians faced barriers resulting from structural vulnerabilities like incarceration and housing insecurity that can increase propensity for moral injuries [1,16,21]. These moral injuries occur due to witnessing, acting, or being unable to act in ways that align with a provider's core beliefs about how clinical care should be practiced and delivered [16]. This case underscores how structurally driven failures are embedded into institutions via deservingness and futility, resulting in morally injurious events for treating clinicians [9,24,25]

4. Implications

Adam's case demonstrates the need for three types of structural health interventions:

1. Restorative justice, community-based reentry programs, and housing as welfare medicine: Punitive justice and hyper-incarceration in the United States is a racist and anti-immigrant complex [26]. Restorative justice [26] and public investment in community building services [18] that may have prevented Adam from being incarcerated are necessary structural and preventive measures.

2. Increased harm reduction services across healthcare especially, penal medicine: Adam repeatedly mentioned the lack of support he received upon release from prison, especially for his substance use. This only emphasizes the need for harm-reduction-based care during the re-entry period, which is a particularly challenging time and a major missed opportunity for intervention.

3. Equitable institutional protocols (contrary to ambiguous guidelines) to treat clinical conditions like IDU-IE that disproportionately impact structurally vulnerable patients: Developing these protocols and guidelines with structurally vulnerable patient populations at the center is imperative for both patients and providers. To provide patient-centered care, protocols must include lived experience. For providers, equitable guidelines may reduce the risk of moral injury.

5. Conclusions

Adam and his physicians underscore how reframing care to focus on patient-centered approaches is a multidimensional approach to mitigating clinician moral injury. A patient-centered approach to medicine that develops interventions for structurally vulnerable patients via clinical, welfare, and penal medicine is a key step towards addressing structural moral injury. Some of the intersecting effects of structural drivers like housing, incarceration, and a lack of programmatic support with ambiguity surrounding treatment guidelines for patients like Adam can be addressed on an institutional level. Consequently, targeted structural and institutional-level approaches that prioritize the wellbeing of Adam and other patients in similar circumstances may prevent clinicians from experiencing barriers to care provision. These can range from MOUD access to family visitation for incarcerated patients. In hospital settings, these would necessitate developing protocols to streamline care of incarcerated patients from the standpoint of what is medically necessitated and medically indicated, as well as identifying key barriers to care for incarcerated patients and leveraging institutional resources to address them.

Funding: This study received funding support from NIDA, grant #RO1DA046049, and the Institute for Addiction Science Pilot Grant Award, University of Southern California—PG1033682.

Conflicts of Interest: The authors declare no conflicts of interest.

Abbreviations

DVT	Deep vein thrombosis
ED	Emergency department
EM	Emergency medicine
IDU-IE	Injection-drug-use-related infective endocarditis
MOUD	Medications for opioid use disorder
PTSD	Post-traumatic stress disorder

References

1. Seim, J.; DiMario, A. City of Gauze: Medicine and the Governance of Urban Poverty. *Soc. Probl.* **2023**, spad041. [CrossRef]
2. Alsan, M.; Yang, C.S.; Jolin, J.R.; Tu, L.; Rich, J.D. Health care in U.S. correctional facilities—A limited and threatened constitutional right. *N. Engl. J. Med.* **2023**, *388*, 847–852. [CrossRef] [PubMed]
3. Sawyer, W.; Wagner, P.; Mass Incarceration: The Whole Pie 2024. Prison Policy Initiative. Available online: https://www.prisonpolicy.org/reports/pie2024.html (accessed on 30 June 2024).

4. Karandinos, G.; Bourgois, P. The structural violence of hyperincarceration—A 44-year-old man with back pain. *N. Engl. J. Med.* **2019**, *380*, 205–209. [CrossRef] [PubMed]
5. Bourgois, P.; Holmes, S.M.; Sue, K.; Quesada, J. Structural vulnerability: Operationalizing the concept to address health disparities in clinical care. *Acad. Med.* **2017**, *92*, 299–307. [CrossRef] [PubMed]
6. Farmer, P.; Nizeye, B.; Stulac, S.; Keshavjee, S. Structural violence and clinical medicine. In *Understanding and Applying Medical Anthropology*; Bourgois, P., Holmes, S.M., Sue, K., Quesada, J., Eds.; Routledge: London, UK, 2016; pp. 336–343.
7. Klein, D.E.; Lima, J.M. The prison industrial complex as a commercial determinant of health. *Am. J. Public Health* **2021**, *111*, 1750–1752. [CrossRef] [PubMed]
8. Tiako, M.J.N.; Hong, S.B.; Bin Mahmood, S.U.M.; Mori, M.; Mangi, A.; Yun, J.; Juthani-Mehta, M.; Geirsson, A. Inconsistent addiction treatment for patients undergoing cardiac surgery for injection drug use-associated infective endocarditis. *J. Addict. Med.* **2020**, *14*, e350–e354. [CrossRef] [PubMed]
9. Hayden, M.; Moore, A. Attitudes and Approaches Towards Repeat Valve Surgery in Recurrent Injection Drug Use-associated Infective Endocarditis: A Qualitative Study. *J. Addict. Med.* **2020**, *14*, 217–223. [CrossRef] [PubMed]
10. Schranz, A.; Barocas, J.A. Infective endocarditis in persons who use drugs: Epidemiology, current management, and emerging treatments. *Infect. Dis. Clin.* **2020**, *34*, 479–493.
11. Grella, C.E.; Ostile, E.; Scott, C.K.; Dennis, M.; Carnavale, J. A scoping review of barriers and facilitators to implementation of medications for treatment of opioid use disorder within the criminal justice system. *Int. J. Drug Policy* **2020**, *81*, 102768. [CrossRef] [PubMed]
12. Pettersson, G.B.; Hussain, S.T. Current AATS guidelines on surgical treatment of infective endocarditis. *Ann. Cardiothorac. Surg.* **2019**, *8*, 630–644. [CrossRef] [PubMed]
13. Salhi, R.; Macias-Konstantopoulos, W.L.; Ryus, C.R. From the Editors—Future Directions to Strengthen the Emergency Department Safety Net. *West. J. Emerg. Med.* **2023**, *24*, 919–920. [CrossRef] [PubMed]
14. Centers for Medicare and Medicaid Services. Emergency Medical Treatment & Labor Act (EMTALA). 6 September 2023. Available online: https://www.cms.gov/medicare/regulations-guidance/legislation/emergency-medical-treatment-labor-act (accessed on 30 June 2024).
15. Zhang, Q.; Mu, M.C.; He, Y.; Cai, Z.L.; Li, Z.C. Burnout in emergency medicine physicians: A meta-analysis and systematic review. *Medicine*, 2020; 99, e21462.
16. Norman, S.B.; Maguen, S. Va.gov: Veterans Affairs. Moral Injury. 20 April 2020. Available online: https://www.ptsd.va.gov/professional/treat/cooccurring/moral_injury.asp (accessed on 8 December 2021).
17. Stensrud, R.H.; Gilbride, D.D.; Bruinekool, R.M. The childhood to prison pipeline: Early childhood trauma as reported by a prison population. *Rehabil. Couns. Bull.* **2019**, *62*, 195–208. [CrossRef]
18. Henry, B.F. Adverse experiences, mental health, and substance use disorders as social determinants of incarceration. *J. Community Psychol.* **2020**, *48*, 744–762. [CrossRef] [PubMed]
19. Gonzalez, J.M.R.; Connell, N.M. Mental health of prisoners: Identifying barriers to mental health treatment and medication continuity. *Am. J. Public Health* **2014**, *104*, 2328–2333. [CrossRef] [PubMed]
20. Curran, J.; Saloner, B.; Winkelman, T.N.; Alexander, G.C. Estimated use of prescription medications among individuals incarcerated in jails and state prisons in the US. *JAMA Health Forum* **2023**, *4*, e230482. [CrossRef] [PubMed]
21. DiMario, A. To Punish, Parent, or Palliate: Governing Urban Poverty through Institutional Failure. *Am. Sociol. Rev.* **2022**, *87*, 860–888. [CrossRef]
22. Hansen, H.; Bourgois, P.; Drucker, E. Pathologizing poverty: New forms of diagnosis, disability, and structural stigma under welfare reform. *Soc. Sci. med.* **2014**, *103*, 76–83. [CrossRef]
23. Muncan, B.; Kim, E.K.; Amabile, A.; Weimer, M.B.; Nguemeni Tiako, M.J.; Vallabhajosyula, P.; Kalogeropoulos, A.P.; Geirsson, A. Cardiac surgeons' perspectives and practices regarding people who use drugs: A scoping review. *J. Card. Surg.* 2022; 37, 630–639.
24. Griffin, B.J.; Purcell, N.; Burkman, K.; Litz, B.T.; Bryan, C.J.; Schmitz, M.; Villierme, C.; Walsh, J.; Maguen, S. Moral injury: An integrative review. *J. Trauma. Stress* **2019**, *32*, 350–362. [CrossRef]
25. Dean, W.; Talbot, S.G. Hard hits of distress. *J. Pediatr. Rehabil. Med.* **2020**, *13*, 3–5. [CrossRef] [PubMed]
26. González, T. Restorative Justice Diversion as a Structural Health Intervention in the Criminal Legal System. *J. Crim. Law Criminol.* **2023**, *113*, 541–591.

MDPI AG
Grosspeteranlage 5
4052 Basel
Switzerland
Tel.: +41 61 683 77 34

Healthcare Editorial Office
E-mail: healthcare@mdpi.com
www.mdpi.com/journal/healthcare

www.ingramcontent.com/pod-product-compliance
Lightning Source LLC
Chambersburg PA
CBHW062101220926
51850CB00010B/2853
9783725857517